Patient-Focused Healing

Nancy Moore
Henrietta Komras

Foreword by Leland R. Kaiser

Patient-Focused Healing

Integrating Caring and Curing
in Health Care

 Jossey-Bass Publishers
San Francisco

Substantial discounts on bulk quantities of Jossey-Bass books
are available to corporations, professional associations, and other
organizations. For details and discount information, contact the
special sales department at Jossey-Bass Inc., Publishers.
(415) 433-1740; Fax (415) 433-0499.

For sales outside the United States, contact Maxwell Macmillan
International Publishing Group, 866 Third Avenue, New York,
New York 10022.

Manufactured in the United States of America

The paper used in this book is acid-free and meets the
State of California requirements for recycled paper
(50 percent recycled waste, including 10 percent
10% POST
CONSUMER
WASTE   postconsumer waste), which are the strictest guidelines
for recycled paper currently in use in the United States.

The ink in this book is either soy- or vegetable-based and during the
printing process emits fewer than half the volatile organic compounds
(VOCs) emitted by petroleum-based ink.

Library of Congress Cataloging-in-Publication Data

Moore, Nancy, date.
    Patient-focused healing : integrating caring and curing in health
care / Nancy Moore, Henrietta Komras.
        p.   cm. — (The Jossey-Bass health series)
    Includes bibliographical references and index.
    ISBN 1-55542-584-4 (alk. paper)
    1. Health services administration.   2. Medical personnel and
patient.   3. Medical care—Philosophy.   I. Komras, Henrietta, date.
    II. Title.   III. Series.
    [DNLM: 1. Holistic Health.   2. Hospital Administration.
3. Quality of Health Care.   WX 153 M825p 1993]
RA971.M566   1993
362.1′1—dc20
DNLM/DLC
for Library of Congress   93-4218
                                                                        CIP

FIRST EDITION
HB Printing   10 9 8 7 6 5 4 3 2 1   *Code 9385*

The Jossey-Bass
Health Series

Contents

Foreword

It is a distinct pleasure for me to write the foreword for this ground-breaking book on patient-focused care. I am well acquainted with both of the authors and have a high regard for their work. Nancy Moore is an experienced bedside nurse as well as an accomplished nurse executive. Henrietta Komras is a nationally recognized independent health care consultant. Moore and Komras work in the "trenches" every day, which shows in their compassion, wisdom, and experience.

The strength of this work shows in the combined talents of its authors. Concept and practice are integrally blended, and real-life examples abound. Key practice-oriented tools include helpful checklists, descriptions of innovative patient-focused sites, listings of resources, and an extensive review of the literature. In many ways this book is a handbook or user's manual, offering a wealth of ideas regarding implementation strategies along with useful contacts, including phone numbers! To find such a quantity of worthwhile material between two covers is unusual, and I know of no other book that puts all this information together as does *Patient-Focused Healing*.

CEOs will be interested in this book because it provides a solid introduction to the subject of patient-focused care and gives excellent examples of successful practical programs. The book is filled with helpful ideas about implementing patient-focused programs in traditional medical care organizations.

Direct-care providers such as physicians and nurses will also benefit from the authors' innovative approaches. The shifting paradigm in health care is well illustrated in the changing relationships among providers, patients, families, and communities. Doctors and nurses have traditionally been the center of action in hospitals. Now, patients and families are of central importance. In the past, patients were expected to adapt to the routines of the hospital. Presently, hospitals and ambulatory care centers are being designed to address the needs and interests of patients and their families and communities.

This new mode of patient care requires nothing short of a revolution in institutional mind-set. However, many health care facilities have not yet changed their approach. *Patient-Focused Healing* will help those managing and staffing such facilities better understand what is required for survival in this turbulent era.

Trustees and financial managers will also benefit from this book. In these changing times, governing boards require a new orientation to patient care, and financial managers must better understand what lies on "the other side of the numbers." Change will not be easy for either group. Patient-focused healing is part of the new vision of health care in the United States, and for this reason, hospital trustees must demand a patient focus, and financial managers must realize its importance to long-term economic survival. Patients will patronize those hospitals with the highest clinical standards of care, the lowest costs, and the best patient-care environments. This rigorous set of survival criteria will be mandated by national health reform and changing customer expectations.

One of the core beliefs of total quality management (TQM) is that health care facilities should meet or exceed customer expectations. In the next seven years, patient-focused healing will become the norm in our hospitals and a key element in customer expectations. Once considered service industries, hospitals are rapidly becoming information industries and will soon evolve into experiential industries. The patient-focused healing model provides the best all-around patient and family experience and offers a better way of delivering services. This model provides a unique view of information handling, involving as it does the patient and family in medical decision making and record keeping.

For the next few years most of our nation's hospitals will be involved in restructuring efforts. Work redesign is essential to meet the new requirements of integrated delivery networks, capitation, and managed care. However, redesign is also necessary to provide better healing environments for patients and their family members. This book is the definitive work on creating healing environments through patient-focused care.

Denver, Colorado   Leland R. Kaiser
August 1993   *president, Kaiser & Associates*
associate professor,
Graduate Program in Health Administration
University of Colorado at Denver

Preface

> The year [2000] is operating like a powerful magnet on
> humanity, reaching down into the 1990's and intensifying
> the decade. It is amplifying emotions, accelerating change,
> heightening awareness, and compelling us to reexamine
> ourselves, our values, and our institutions.
>
> John Naisbitt and Patricia Aburdene,
> *Megatrends 2000**

As we are poised at the dawn of a new century, health
care is undergoing a major crisis. Members of the health care
profession are looking within and asking, What business are we
in? There is a pressing need by everyone in the health care community to rediscover values and reconnect with the original
mission of health care. It is the premise of this book that the
fundamental "business" of health care is to set the stage for and
to create the environment that supports an individual's own
healing process and that encourages the interaction and partnership of patients, families, and professional caregivers.

Traditionally, hospitals have designed their operations
around technology and the needs of the special interests of health
care professionals. This orientation has resulted in a provider
focus rather than a patient-focused approach to the delivery of
health care services. This approach has been neither efficient
nor cost-effective, as one can easily see when one considers that
the United States spent $800 billion on health care in 1992, with
an estimated projected expense of $1.6 trillion by the end of
the decade. Despite the enormous amount spent on health care,

---

*John Naisbitt and Patricia Aburdene, *Megatrends 2000*, © 1990, Megatrends Ltd., represented by William Morrow and Co., Inc.

we have failed to solve our most vexing health problems, such as cancer, chronic degenerative disease, and substance abuse.

We believe that the survival and excellence of health care in this country depend on two key strategies: introduction of a holistic approach to healing that integrates body, mind, and spirit, and restructuring of the delivery of services by placing patients and their needs at the center of the health care mission. We believe implementing patient-focused care, a concept that combines these two strategies, will decrease hospital costs and improve the quality and continuity of care. As a result, physicians, nurses, and other caregivers will be more satisfied than they are now, and consumers will regain their confidence in our health care system.

Patient-Focused Healing presents an overview of the elements of patient-focused care and offers practical suggestions for implementing this approach. Throughout the book we draw on the experience of hospitals that have implemented patient-focused care as well as the work of visionary writers, researchers, and leaders, including Leland R. Kaiser, health care futurist; Dolores Krieger, developer of therapeutic touch; Angelica Thieriot, creator of Planetree; Philip Lathrop, prominent consultant in operational restructuring; Roger Ulrich, design researcher; W. Edwards Deming, noted quality expert, as well as others who have influenced our vision of the future of health care. We also offer our personal experience and observations, drawn from our many years in health care. Our approach combines factual reporting with passion and dedication to making a change in the health care field.

We are personally involved and concerned with the future of health care in this country. We believe that health care is presently operating in a crisis mode: a time of shrinking reimbursement, intense competition, rapid technological advances, and increasing consumer dissatisfaction. According to a recent survey, two out of every five Americans view health care as "the biggest problem facing the U.S. today, outranking education and crime" (Clements, 1993, p. 4). Because health care has failed to address people's concerns, a solution is now being sought by the federal government.

President Clinton's forthcoming reform plan is likely to rely on three major concepts: universal access, managed competition, and global budgeting/cost control. In managed competition, the foundation of the proposed reform, the federal government facilitates the establishment of large health insurance–purchasing cooperatives. These cooperatives will accept competitive bids from multiprovider health networks. Theoretically, this system promotes competition among health plans, encouraging bidding for contracts, thus reducing costs and improving quality. With this system, the federal government would establish a minimum level of benefits and regulate the provider networks through state-level or regional health boards (Sandrick, 1993). As a result, hospitals and providers, including physicians, would be married in an effort to meet consumers' primary health care need: quality health care at the lowest cost.

We believe that the structure of hospital operations and the predominantly technological focus of traditional health care have created a distance between health care practitioners and the people they serve. In our opinion, health care has, unfortunately, lost touch with its primary purpose: to create a healing environment where both patients and health care professionals can work together to heal the body, mind, and spirit of all individuals who come seeking healing. We need to reconnect with this purpose. It is at the core of the mission of the first healers: the physicians of ancient Greece who understood that the root of the word *heal* comes from the word *holy* — to make whole. They understood what we may have lost touch with, that to heal one must integrate the resources of the whole person — body, mind, and spirit — and all these components must work in harmony. Florence Nightingale echoes this mission in *Notes on Nursing* (1946 [1859], pp. 74–75): "It is often thought that medicine is the curative process. It is no such thing: medicine is the surgery of functions. . . . Surgery removes the bullet out of the limb, which is the obstruction to cure, but nature heals the wound. So it is with medicine: . . . [medicine] assists nature to remove the obstruction, but nothing more. And what nursing has to do in either case, is to put the patient in the best condition for nature to act upon him."

This book is about our belief that the purpose of health care is "to put the patient in the best condition for nature to act upon him." In our vision for health care, we look beyond the patient. Individuals do not exist in isolation: they are members ɔf families, social groups, work groups, communities, and nations; they live in constant interaction with their environment. For example, to help a patient with chronic obstructive lung disease without addressing the smog-filled air he breathes is foolhardy; to repair the broken bones of an abused child without tending to the dynamics of the family situation is criminal negligence.

If ever there was a time for leadership in creating a healing environment and rededicating ourselves to the healing mission of health care, the time is now. We believe that health care leaders can turn this time of crisis into a time of opportunity. Health care can fulfill this vital role if it chooses to adopt this mission. We invite our readers to critique our ideas, to expand on them, and to join us in envisioning a new mission for health care.

Many books written on health care focus on purely economic problems like the crisis of access to health care and escalating costs. Many also focus on organizational development in health care and address specific elements such as improving the efficiency of operating rooms or decreasing the waiting time for tests. Although these are important concerns, this book is unique because of its global approach; it encompasses many elements connected by the common thread of placing the patient at the center of the hospital's mission. Rather than concentrating on specific aspects of hospital operations, *Patient-Focused Healing* contains a systems perspective based on the principle that to solve problems in health care we need to examine the whole system as well as its parts. This book presents a new paradigm that replaces a provider focus with a patient-focused approach.

Health care is indeed operating in a crisis mode; however, crisis can be seen in two ways. The Chinese character for crisis, *we chai*, combines the symbol for danger with the symbol for opportunity (Dai, 1970). Therefore, the ancient wisdom of the Chinese can allow us to see only the danger inherent in any crisis, or it can challenge us to interpret crisis as an opportunity for change. We can change our vision for the mission of health care if we allow ourselves the courage to change. Kaiser echoes this challenge when he states, "What a wonderful time to be in the healthcare industry! Everything is falling apart" (quoted in Ryan, 1991, p. 1). This book is unique in that it focuses on the opportunities available to health care if we choose to focus on the challenge rather than be intimidated by the danger.

Audience

The primary audience for this book is hospital administrators. We have chosen this audience because it is their role to provide the visionary leadership needed to design patient-focused health care. This book addresses the problems and challenges ahead and provides ideas and suggestions for making the needed changes. In addition, it is an excellent resource for nurses, physicians, patients, policy makers, and the host of other professionals dedicated to health care. These professionals must work together if health care is to undergo a transformation and to achieve its full potential.

Overview of the Contents

This book begins with a conceptual framework for understanding the elements of patient-focused care and explains why this is rapidly becoming the preferred model for health care as we move into the twenty-first century. This book also outlines practical strategies for implementing patient-focused care and includes many examples and suggestions based on the experience of those involved with these concepts. In each chapter, we describe the fundamental concepts of each element of patient-focused care, including real-life examples, and, wherever possible, we provide supporting research. We close the book with a summary of our vision of health care's future and practical advice for how to become involved in the process of transformation.

Chapter One compares the traditional care model with the patient-focused model. We introduce the concept of patient-focused care by outlining the major themes to be explored in the book: creating healing environments, involving patients in their own care by emphasizing patient education, and restructuring hospital operations to increase efficiency and decrease costs. We summarize some of the social trends that are shaping the future of health care and the impact that these trends will have. These trends point to the need to transform our health care institutions so that they have a patient-focused approach. Finally, we explore the basic components of patient-focused care.

Chapter Two examines the crucial topic of the effect of patient-focused care on the bottom line: How does this model affect costs and quality of care? We begin by documenting the staggering costs and inefficiency that result from the traditional, highly centralized structure of hospital operations. We then explain the advantages of restructuring operations and decentralizing patient care. At the end of this chapter we document the significant improvements that occur as a result of these changes and how they translate into such benefits as decreased costs, reduced errors, and increased patient satisfaction.

Chapter Three presents the case for putting healing back into health care. After defining the concept of healing and its implications for patient care, we examine the vital role of patient and family empowerment. In this section, we present research supporting this vital therapeutic intervention and offer examples from hospitals applying these concepts. We next present evidence that the manner in which caregivers interact with patients affects the quality of their healing as we explore "therapeutic presence." Then we explore mind/body therapies that have proven themselves in enhancing patient empowerment and healing. Finally, we look at how the physical environment can be harnessed to enhance healing through the use of patient-centered architecture and design.

Chapter Four addresses the practical aspects of implementing patient-focused care based on the experience of pioneering hospitals. We begin by explaining the importance of beginning the process by assessing the unique characteristics and requirements of each setting. We then discuss the role of consultants and offer some useful guidelines for choosing them. We next present three principles to guide the process — systems thinking, staff involvement, and visionary leadership — and describe steps in the transformation process. Case studies of hospitals that have been through patient-focused restructuring illustrate successful transformations. We conclude the chapter with guidelines for managing the emotional side of the change process and a review of the problems and lessons learned.

Chapter Five explores the role of the health care team in the patient-focused hospital. We begin by looking at the problems generated by the present system of care delivery and the negative effects of this approach on physicians, nursing staff, ancillary staff, and support staff. Then, after exploring two major concerns—the decreasing supply of professionals and the need to increase quality while decreasing costs—we present some promising new care approaches. These exciting new models include nursing case management, the Nursing Network, primary care, the Professionally Advanced Care Team, and a variety of nurse-extender models. Finally, we explore the implications of patient-centered care for management and describe two examples of team empowerment: shared governance and shared leadership.

Chapter Six presents strategies for promoting patient-focused healing through design and architecture. We examine considerations in patient-focused design: how to help people find their way around hospitals, how to promote physical and psychological comfort, and how to meet both privacy needs and the need for social contact. We also explore other elements of design such as lighting, the use of color and artwork, and the importance of integrating the presence of nature. We continue the chapter by examining the design principles necessary for specific spaces such as waiting and reception areas, diagnostic and treatment areas, patient rooms, and specialized units including rehabilitation centers, pediatric facilities, birthing units, and hospices. We conclude with guidelines for choosing health care design teams.

Chapter Seven presents strategies for implementing healing health care. We begin by exploring the concept that health care is a human service as we present strategies for enhancing therapeutic presence. This section suggests building hospital culture through development of the organization's unique mythology and proposes a variety of other strategies, including employee-wellness programs and team development. Next, we focus on patient and family empowerment by offering strategies that encourage active participation and learning as well as personal involvement in the healing process. In addition, we include practical suggestions for gaining physician support for and staff commitment to patient-education programs. We outline strategies for implementing nontraditional therapies. We continue with guidelines for creating a customer-driven organization and a culture that thrives on change. We close this chapter with a summary of barriers to implementation and lessons learned.

Chapter Eight offers a visionary overview of some possibilities for the evolution of health care as we approach the twenty-first century. We begin with the opinions of health care leaders about the future of health care, based on a survey of those leaders. Then we present our vision for a new era of health care and explore three forces shaping a new view: general systems theory, a model of the learning society, and medicine that incorporates high-tech and alternative methods. Next, we take an imaginative journey to explore what new health care might look like as we change its nature and its relationship to a changing society and a changing world. We conclude with an invitation to our readers to join us in defining this new era.

Chapter Nine tells how to become involved and where to begin. We address the needs of four broad categories of readers: health care consumers, hospital administrators, nurses and other health care professionals, and physicians. In each section we offer specific strategies tailored to the unique needs of each of these groups. We close this chapter with a reminder that in order to truly transform health care, we need to recognize that this task involves everyone and that the goal is to create a system that enhances the health of all people.

The Resources Directory at the end of the book lists a variety of resources on patient-focused care and healing health care for readers who want to continue learning about these exciting trends. These resources include books, journals, organizations and associations, audiovisual resources, computer networks, consultants, and places to visit.

Acknowledgments

We express our gratitude and appreciation to our spouses, Lin Moore and Robert Sternberg, and to the friends who contributed the wisdom, insight, and energy that made writing this book possible. We also want to give special recognition to the many people of St. Charles Medical Center of Bend, Oregon, who supported us throughout this process and are model providers of health care that heals as well as cures.

August 1993   Nancy Moore
                                                 Bend, Oregon

                                                 Henrietta Komras
                                                 St. Louis, Missouri

The Authors

NANCY MOORE, RN, MS, CNA, LPC, is Healing Health-care project director and manager of Mental Health Services at St. Charles Medical Center in Bend, Oregon. She received her R.N. degree (1966) in nursing from Bethesda Hospital School of Nursing and her B.A. degree (1977) in psychology and literature from Antioch College, as well as her M.S. degree (1989) in counseling from Oregon State University. Currently she is a Ph.D. candidate in healing health care at Greenwich University, where Leland Kaiser is her faculty mentor.

With over a quarter of a century as a practicing hospital nurse and manager, Moore has a rich knowledge of the practice of health care in this country. She is listed in the National Distinguished Registry in Nursing (1988) and Who's Who in American Nursing (1990–1993). Also she is a member of Kaiser & Associates Consulting Services Network. Her publications include articles in *Nursing Management* magazine and the *Healing Healthcare Network Newsletter.* She has presented papers on topics such as therapeutic touch, therapeutic presence, caring for the whole person, and counseling skills for the caregiver.

HENRIETTA KOMRAS is a management consultant and nationally known speaker and trainer specializing in the health care field. She owns her own company, Komras & Associates, Inc., based in St. Louis, Missouri. She received her B.A. degree (1973) in communication and psychology from Antioch College and her M.A. degree (1977) in educational technology from Concordia University in Canada. Currently she is a Ph.D. candidate in management at Columbia Pacific University.

Komras works with hospitals across the country and has led workshops on topics such as empowerment for health care managers, performance management, patient-focused care, and self-esteem. She has spoken before many hospital associations and professional groups and has won numerous sales awards for her work in marketing training programs for health care clients across the country. Her articles have been published in magazines and newsletters, including the *ASHHRA* (American Society of Healthcare Human Resources Association) *Newsletter.* She is a member of Kaiser & Associates Consulting Services Network. She has extensive experience in organizational development and has consulted with many organizations about organizational change and management development.

Patient-Focused Healing

Chapter 1

When Health Care Centers on the Patient

We must learn to balance the wonders of technology with the spiritual demands of our human nature.

John Naisbitt, *Megatrends*

A patient is kept waiting for a routine x-ray for over two hours.

A nurse awakens a patient at 6:00 A.M. to give him his medication. It is hospital policy to give medications at that time.

A patient is wheeled across the entire hospital for a series of laboratory tests.

A patient wants to discuss alternative forms of treatment with her physician. She is told that the physician has no time to see her.

A patient wants to find out more about his condition. The nurse informs him that he will be well taken care of so he does not really need all that information.

A patient is perplexed by the number of personnel she has been in contact with during the week she has been in the hospital. She has seen sixty to seventy different faces since the day she arrived.

These types of episodes still occur on a daily basis in hospitals across the United States; however, this kind of treatment is not conducive to consumer satisfaction.

If we ask who or what is at the center of the hospital experience, we can arrive at several possible answers: the policies and procedures of the hospital, medical technology, the physician, or some other aspect of hospital operations. Unfortunately, the

1

recipient of all our care, the patient, is often not at the center of our concerns.

Now, let's imagine a different situation. A patient is asleep in her comfortable hospital room. Light is streaming in from the window, and soft music is playing in the background. Soft colors and indirect lighting permeate the rooms and the hallways of this hospital. The room has woodwork, rather than stainless steel, the sheets and covers are a soft pastel color rather than white, and there is artwork on the wall. All the surroundings are designed with peace and harmony in mind.

In addition to its appearance, other features of the hospital are designed for efficiency and comfort. A bedside computer terminal is used for documentation, the scheduling of ancillary services, and the ordering of supplies. The traditional high counter of the nurses' station has been replaced with one that allows for free interaction between patients and the nursing staff. Rather than having carts wheeled around in the hallways, "patient servers" (compact storage units) are built into each room to provide everything needed for patient care including medical supplies, nursing notes, and records. The hallways are quiet and subdued rather than hectic thoroughfares because ancillary services, such as admissions, laboratory work, and radiology work, have been decentralized.

Everything in this hospital is designed to help the patient feel as if she were at home rather than in an institution. The serving of food and the dispensing of medication are scheduled according to patient preference rather than for the convenience of the staff. Some floors in this hospital even have kitchenettes so that the patient or her family can prepare a home-cooked meal or keep favorite snacks in the refrigerator. A patient lounge with videotapes and audiotapes provides entertainment and relaxation and a much needed respite from the monotony of always being in the same room.

Emphasis in this hospital is on patient involvement and education. Patients and family members are taught some routine patient-care procedures — an important benefit for all patients because hospital stays have decreased in length and, therefore, many patients go home still requiring care.

Genesis and Major Themes
of Patient-Focused Care

This is not some utopian fantasy or a description of an ideal hospital in the distant future. Elements of this model of patient-focused care are already in place in some leading hospitals across the country. Driven by consumer demand, rising costs, and staff dissatisfaction, health care providers are redefining the mission of health care and reexamining some of the assumptions on which traditional hospital procedures are based. A paradigm shift is taking place—a shift from a provider focus to a patient-centered focus. This shift is taking place because it has become evident that the hospital of the past, with its highly complex, centralized, and bureaucratic method of delivering services to patients, can no longer continue to exist. In order to increase productivity and improve customer satisfaction, health care providers will have to rectify the built-in inefficiencies of the existing model.

Planetree

We will begin our exploration of patient-focused care by examining one of the pioneering organizations with this focus, the Planetree unit at California Pacific Medical Center in San Francisco. Founded in 1978 by Angelica Thieriot, it was one of the first experiments in empowering patients by involving them in their own care and providing them with the information and education necessary to make decisions about their own healing process. Interestingly, the founder of Planetree was not a professional in the health care field. She was a health care consumer. Here is her story.

"I felt as though I'd lost my status as an adult . . . and was treated with disdain and annoyance, even ignored. I never saw the same doctor twice and if I asked any questions, I was told I would have to ask my doctor. . . . I was shocked by the bungling and constantly changing staff. At one point, I was left slumped over in a wheelchair outside x-ray for 45 minutes with a fever of 107 degrees" (quoted in Jenna, 1986a, p. 9). According to Thieriot, her own physicians were unwilling to give her information about her diagnosis and about the treatments that they proposed.

Understandably, she was upset at not being able to participate in important decisions regarding her care. Ironically, her ailment was never diagnosed properly, apparently because of a laboratory mix-up. Thieriot was also uncomfortable with the odd, impersonal nature of the physical environment. This aspect of her hospital experience was no better than the level of personal care. "I was in a horrible tiny room with a view of the wall. Except for an orchid which my mother-in-law gave me, there was nothing in the room that could give me any solace" (p. 10).

Thieriot founded Planetree as a response to the unsatisfactory care she received while being hospitalized. Based on this experience and her conviction that such treatment was not necessary, Thieriot began to develop a vision of a hospital that would emphasize patient involvement, patient education, and a healing, homelike atmosphere. From this vision, the dream of Planetree slowly became reality, and the unit has become a model for hospitals across the country.

Thieriot's negative experience occurred in a health care organization with a provider focus rather than a patient-centered focus. In this type of environment, the policies of the organization and the convenience of the staff determine the way care is provided. Patients are often treated as cases rather than as individuals, as helpless children whose role is to obey the "experts" and follow their orders. Patients are expected to conform to the rules and policies of the institution and do as they are told. As one patient remarked: "It seems that when patients enter a hospital, they leave their adult status at the door" (quoted in Jenna, 1986a, p. 8). Because patients are made to feel like children, they soon come to depend on the "adults" to make them feel better. In such a state of powerlessness, most patients will not question their caregivers and will not complain for fear of antagonizing them.

Two Themes

Patient-focused care is a multipronged approach that combines many different elements. However, two major themes emerge:

one is the need to create a healing environment and to involve patients in their own healing process; the other is the need to restructure hospital operations to increase efficiency, provide continuity of care, and reduce waiting time.

One model of patient-focused care is based on the premise that to increase efficiency and to improve service we need to restructure hospital operations. Such restructuring involves decentralizing the hospital so that we bring services to the patient rather than bringing the patient to the services. The other patient-focused model is based on the belief that patients can contribute to their own healing process. In this model, the role of the hospital is to provide an optimum healing environment for body, mind, and spirit.

One model focuses on structure and delivery systems, while the other focuses on empowering patients and creating a healing environment. These are two sides of the same coin. Combining both models will result in a fundamental shift in the way hospitals are organized and in the patient's hospital experience.

Trends Supporting the
Patient-Focused Movement

Before examining the patient-focused model in detail, we will outline the trends shaping the shift from the traditional provider-focused model to patient-focused care. As we approach the year 2000, it is evident that we are experiencing rapid change and upheaval. These changes are already having a tremendous impact on many institutions in our society. The past several decades have been an era of transition; established paradigms have been challenged, and new forms of organization and life-style have emerged. Transformation is occurring at an astounding rate as traditions are questioned and we realize that we need to redesign and restructure existing organizations.

Health care has been one of the institutions undergoing transformation; consumers have asserted their autonomy and withdrawn their former unquestioned loyalty from what many now consider to be an authoritarian system. In this age of self-help movements, of networks, and of empowerment, consumers find that the health care system is no longer meeting their needs. Both providers and consumers are seeking ways to revitalize the practice of medicine in this country.

Leland Kaiser, prominent speaker and health care futurist, has characterized the decade of the 1980s as the whitewater era in health care and believes that the 1990s will be the period of "going over the falls" (Kaiser, 1991e, p. 73). When confronting this time of crisis in health care, we can choose between a pessimistic view of the future or an optimistic belief that this can be a period of opportunity. The future will be what we make it: it is ours to choose.

Patient as Customer

One of the most important trends in health care today is a recognition of the needs and demands of an increasingly educated and sophisticated consumer. During the 1980s, the number of choices available to consumers grew tremendously. This increase in choices entailed a shift from a seller's to a buyer's market in health care. As a result we must redefine our mission and place the patient at the center of our concerns because the consumer, not the institution or specialist, makes decisions about health care (Zemke, 1987, p. 42).

Research shows that consumers are taking an active and informed part in determining their own care. Today, 70 percent of patients indicate that they make the decision regarding where to go for treatment. Although many patients do follow the recommendation of their physicians, most are inclined to be assertive about their needs. "There clearly is a new consumer out there, one who is willing to change doctors . . . to get health-care delivered to them the way they want it delivered" (Zemke, 1987, p. 42).

Patients evaluate their care on how they are treated: whether they are kept waiting, whether they are informed about their treatment, whether caregivers are empathetic and understanding. They base their decisions on the aspects of their treatment that they feel qualified to judge: the room, the food, the admissions process, the questions they are asked, the answers they get to their questions, how hard it is to find a parking place, and whether the caregivers they interact with are friendly.

Consumers assume an adequate level of medical expertise from all health care institutions. The factors that distinguish a health care organization are the quality of human interaction and the environment. Patients want to have access to information, they want to be actively involved, they want to be treated as individuals, they want comfortable surroundings, and they want the staff they interact with to care. Patient-focused care, with its emphasis on involvement and continuity of care, can respond to all these concerns.

"Prosumer" Society

Closely related to the trend of patient-as-customer is the rise of what Alvin Toffler calls the "prosumer." In his phophetic book, *The Third Wave,* he described a "progressive blurring of the line that separates producer from consumer" (Toffler, 1981, p. 267). In a consumer society, Toffler explained, the task of consumption has been totally separated from that of production, making the consumer dependent on the products and expertise of the producer. In contrast, the prosumer society empowers passive consumers and turns them into active participants capable of solving their own problems and doing things for themselves.

One example described by Toffler is the do-it-yourself pregnancy-test kits launched on the market in the 1970s. The availability of such kits was significant in the rise of the prosumer society, according to Toffler, because the kits allowed women to perform for themselves a task previously done for them by others, specifically by doctors and laboratories. It is interesting to note that Toffler used a medical example to illustrate this shift because it shows the health care consumer becoming the involved, empowered health care prosumer. Toffler commented on the growing self-care movement: "The idea that people can and should be more medically self-reliant is a fast rolling new bandwagon. . . . Ordinary people are learning to handle stethoscopes and blood pressure cuffs, administer breast self-examinations and Pap smears, even carry out elementary surgical procedures" (p. 265). Patient-focused care caters to the empowered patient, the prosumer rather than the consumer of health care.

Information Society

In his groundbreaking book, *Megatrends,* Naisbitt (1984) documents the transformation of our society from the Industrial Age to the Information Age. The Industrial Age is based on the manufacture of mass-produced consumer goods and is dependent on the availability of natural resources such as coal and oil. The Information Age is characterized by the growing importance of the service sector of the economy and is fueled by a virtually inexhaustible resource: information.

This major shift has had a profound impact on every aspect of health care, especially on the widespread availability of medical information and knowledge. Such knowledge now belongs to everyone. It is no longer held by the elite few of the medical establishment. Magazines, books, and newspaper articles on medical topics are available to everyone, and major television channels all have their medical segment. Medical professionals are challenged to keep up with their patients' questions about the latest breakthrough as seen on the evening news.

In the Information Age, both patient education and patient involvement need to be stressed. The patient-focused model responds to this need because these two elements are central to its mission of caring.

Self-Help Movement

Another important trend contributing to the need for patient-focused care is the self-help movement. Naisbitt (1984) reports that for years Americans used institutions such as the medical establishment as a buffer against life's harsh realities and mysteries. "We allowed ourselves to act as passive bystanders, handing over to the medical establishment not only the responsibilities it could handle, healing traumatic wounds and grave illnesses, but also the responsibility for our health and well-being. We revered doctors as our society's high priests and denigrated our own instincts. And in response, the medical establishment sought to live up to our misplaced expectations. Placing all their trust in the modern voodoo of drugs and surgery, they practiced their priesthood and we believed" (Naisbitt, 1984, p. 144).

Naisbitt describes three major trends behind the move from institutional help to self-help: new habits that arise out of a newfound responsibility for health—habits such as exercising, reducing fat intake, reducing liquor consumption, and decreasing smoking; self-care in areas that do not require professional help, such as the use of home medical tests; and the triumph of the wellness model, preventive medicine, and holistic care (Naisbitt, 1984, p. 147).

In *The Third Wave,* Toffler also writes about the growing self-help movement. Toffler estimates that over 500,000 groups in the United States help people deal directly with their own problems rather than relying exclusively on the help of experts. The rapid speed with which the self-help movement continues to spread illustrates the fact that consumers are becoming empowered and are asserting their need to have increased control over and input into all aspects of their lives. It illustrates a rejection of the concept of relying on others to solve problems.

The self-help movement has already had a tremendous impact on the attitude of health care consumers. During the 1970s, Americans began to awaken to the harsh reality that no magic pill, no high-tech fix would solve instantly their most vexing health problems, such as addiction, cancer, and chronic degenerative diseases. As consumers began to take increased responsibility for their health habits and life-style, they began to demand to be treated as individuals with physical, emotional, intellectual, and spiritual needs. When the focus was on the institution, the patient got what the institution prescribed. It did not matter what the patient wanted because the "doctor knows best." Most patients, feeling inferior because of their lack of knowledge, hesitated to question why a certain test was prescribed or why they were awakened at 5 A.M. to take a pill.

Today, the role of the physician and hospital has shifted from doing things for people to helping people to do things for themselves. The result is the rise of consumer-driven, patient-focused approaches such as the hospice movement and birthing centers. Patient-focused care responds to this trend by emphasizing patient involvement and patient education.

Holistic Health

The trend toward a holistic approach to health care indicates a shift away from merely treating symptoms to recognizing the integral relationship of body, mind, and spirit. In *The Aquarian Conspiracy*, Ferguson documents a growing movement that views many nontraditional healing systems as complementary to Western medicine. According to Ferguson, the growth of the wellness movement and the gradual acceptance of such techniques as acupuncture, biofeedback, and chiropractic indicate the beginning of a new kind of health care. Ferguson cites evidence for this growing movement and explains that the American consumer has begun to accept the limitations of the "paradigms and practices of western allopathic medicine with its focus on pathology and disease rather than prevention, the destructiveness of . . . surgical remedies and the too-rigid separation of physical and emotional problems" (Ferguson, 1987, p. 263).

In the future, the integration of alternative techniques into the existing Western model of medicine will continue to increase as consumers challenge the existing paradigm. Patient-focused care, with its acceptance of a holistic model of body, mind, and spirit, already embraces the new paradigm. Patient-focused care is responding to this trend by allowing relaxation techniques, visualization, music, and art to be part of the healing process.

Decentralization

Naisbitt (1984) states that large centralized structures are crumbling all across the United States and are being replaced by smaller, more decentralized units. Naisbitt describes decentralization as a shift away from hierarchies to networks, a shift from bureaucratic forms of organization to simpler, more informal networks. According to Naisbitt, this trend is evident in many different areas of society. In politics, for example, the failure of centralized, top-down solutions led to an upsurge in groups demanding participation in decision making. Small political units, such as grass-roots movements, are claiming local authority and taking responsibility for addressing social issues. This same impulse, explains Naisbitt, is evident in crime fighting, where citizens are taking responsibility for their own safety by forming crime-watch groups.

This shift can also be seen in organizational structures, which are changing from being authoritarian, top-down hierarchies to promoting a participative style of management that encourages shared decision making and problem solving. In health care, the downsizing of management has resulted in the need to decentralize authority and empower employees to meet customer needs and solve problems on the job.

Decentralization empowers individuals and diminishes the power of outside authority. Decentralization is part of new models of management and decision making for hospital staff. One example is the shared-governance model, which empowers nurses at all levels to become involved in making decisions that affect the practice of nursing in the hospital. Patient-focused care responds to this trend by emphasizing the involvement of patients as full participants in their own healing process.

Quality-Improvement Movement

One of the major trends in all organizations today, and especially in health care, is quality improvement. Total quality management (TQM) and continuous quality improvement (CQI) are being implemented in most hospitals in the United States. Based on the techniques of Edward Deming, the goal of TQM is to analyze all processes in an organization and discover methods for improving them. The premise behind this technique is that all processes can be improved.

TQM has not always been accepted in the United States. Deming had to go to a foreign country, Japan, to sell his ideas. Americans watched in awe as the stature of the Japanese, under the leadership of Deming, rose in economic and trade areas.

As Americans began to study the success of the Japanese, they were shocked by the simplicity of the method. The Japanese developed their products around their customers' needs (Beckham, 1991). Recognizing that the worker was closest to the customer, they valued the opinions of workers and involved them in decision making and problem solving through such techniques as quality circles and work teams.

Although American industry rediscovered Deming in the early 1980s, health care has only recently joined the national trend toward quality improvement, employee participation, and a true customer-service orientation. For example, in 1990, the Joint Commission on Accreditation of Healthcare Organizations issued revised nursing standards that require the patient to be the center of care.

Quality improvement is based on the concept that offering the highest quality services requires an on-going process of tracking results and measuring them against standards of excellence. This need to examine all existing processes and practices is especially crucial in health care because many of the processes and systems in health care are based on traditions and on procedures that have been in place for many years rather than on evidence that these procedures deliver the best possible service to the customer. The quality-improvement process embraces change and includes an openness to innovation. The need for continuous learning is integral.

Health care has embraced this trend in order to find innovative ways to implement a service philosophy that is customer-driven and inspired by a vision of greatness. Patient-focused care, with its emphasis on redesigning work tasks, eliminating inefficiency, and increasing productivity, is responding to the need for health care to become dedicated to the quality-improvement process.

High Tech and High Touch

Naisbitt (1984) urges us to learn to balance the "material wonders of technology with the spiritual demands of our human nature." He explains that whenever new technology is introduced, there has to be a balancing response that stresses human interaction, what he terms "high touch." "The more high tech, the more high touch is needed" (Naisbitt, 1984, p. 34).

According to Naisbitt, this trend has had a tremendous impact on health care. One example he refers to is the fact that as we introduced the high technology of life-sustaining equipment in our hospitals, there was a corresponding growth in the hospice movement and concern about the quality of death and dying in our hospitals. As a counterbalancing force to the high technology of heart transplants, brain scanners, laser surgery, and CAT scans, medical care is becoming increasingly high touch as staff in hospitals attempt to create a homelike atmosphere. Birthing centers, the hospice movement, and primary nursing are all part of this emphasis on TLC, or tender loving care. Patient-focused care, with its basis in continuity of care and healing environments, is a response to this growing trend.

Changing Workforce

Much documentation supports the changing nature of the workforce in the United States. In addition to being more diverse in ethnic origin and cultural background, today's workforce is more educated and more demanding of employers than it was in the past. Employees today have less of a tendency to devote themselves to their employers and do not automatically give them their unquestioned loyalty. Workers today know that they cannot be guaranteed job security and escalating salaries, so they expect their employers to meet their personal-growth needs in the short run to maintain their loyalty (Leebov and Scott, 1990, p. 3).

Employees today want to make a contribution and find a sense of meaning and purpose in their work. They want to be involved in decision making and problem solving, and they want to be able to use their creativity and initiative. They are not content just to do as they are told; they want to be fully participating members, involved in fulfilling the organization's mission. If these needs are not satisfied, hospitals will not be able to attract and retain loyal, committed, and creative employees.

This trend is affecting the way we need to manage today's health care employee. Satisfaction on the job has decreased substantially for many health care workers, especially in such fields as nursing. Much of this dissatisfaction stems from the alienation and frustration that nurses feel on the job when they spend most of their day on such tasks as documentation, charting, record keeping, and general "paper pushing" rather than on direct patient care. Individuals who entered the nursing profession did not choose this field in order to do paperwork.

Health care needs to respond to this challenge by creating an environment and a culture that allow each employee to contribute fully and to find satisfaction on the job. Patient-focused care includes redesigning jobs so that employees can serve patients effectively and can therefore increase their own satisfaction. For example, when nurses' jobs are redesigned in patient-focused settings, nurses can spend more time in direct patient care rather than on paperwork. As a result, nurses gain increased satisfaction on the job.

Changing Reimbursement Rules

At one time hospitals were reimbursed by third-party payers—insurance companies and government agencies—based on cost. This system ended in October 1983, when the diagnostic-related-grouping (DRG) payment plan went into effect. Since then, hospitals have been reimbursed at a fixed rate based on the diagnosis of the patient.

Under the DRG system, because any procedure, from an appendectomy to childbirth, is reimbursed at a fixed rate, the hospital that performs at or below cost is profitable and succeeds. Hospitals that are unable to keep treatment costs in line with these payment guidelines can easily be out of business. Managed-care plans and employer-partnership plans also present hospitals with the challenge to be cost-effective. Patient-focused care is a positive response to the challenge of containing hospital costs because it increases efficiency and reduces the cost of delivery systems.

Elements of Patient-Focused Care

There are some major differences between the traditional health care model and the patient-focused model. We will examine each of these elements as outlined in the following chart.

Traditional patient care	*Patient-focused model*
Provider focus	Patient at the center
Reliance on experts	Active patient and family involvement
Impersonal atmosphere	Healing environment
Many caregivers	Continuity of care
Centralized services	Decentralization
Specialization	Cross-training to produce multiskilled practitioners
Treatment of symptoms	Holistic approach
Lengthy documentation	Streamlined documentation

Patient at the Center

Patient-focused care is an antidote to the passive, dependent role that patients often play in the modern hospital. Their help-less state is eloquently described by Thompson in his book *The American Replacement of Nature.* "The flesh here [in the hospital] is surrounded with plastic, inserted with tubes, and subjected to radiation and tranquilizing drugs to force it to accept medical confinement and professional processing. . . . The drugged steer in the feedlot and the sick human in the modern hospital are not different cases, for both have lost their freedom, and both are constrained to accept a professionalized approach . . . in a technologically managed institution" (Thompson, 1991, p. 121).

The concept of patient-focused health care is founded on a need to redefine the mission of the health care organization. Within the traditional hospital, the physician reigns supreme and acts as the gatekeeper of the organization. In this setting, the patient's well-being is defined by the physician without much involvement of the patient. The physician is the all-knowing "parent," and the patient is the dependent "child" who must listen to the physician and do what he is told.

In contrast, a patient-focused approach begins with the premise that the patient sets the stage for her own healing or recovery, with the physician, nursing staff, and other caregivers providing needed technical and emotional resources. In this model of patient care, the caregivers are part of a team that includes the patient. Patient education becomes a crucial component, providing patients with information they need. Patients can then intelligently discuss their condition, learn about possible treatments, and participate in decisions about their own care.

Patient Involvement and Education

In the past, there has been much debate about whether to educate patients and involve them in decisions concerning their own course of treatment. Some of the arguments against patient involvement include the fear that the patient may make the wrong decision, that providing patients with detailed information is too time-consuming, and that if patients are informed about the possible side-effects of their medication, this knowledge may contribute to the development of side-effects.

Need for Patient Involvement. Much of the evidence in studies published in major medical journals shows that the opposite is true. This research indicates that patients who are involved in their own medical decisions and knowledgeable actually get well quicker than those who are not involved or knowledgeable (Summers, 1985, p. 55). As a matter of fact, research reports show that the traditional practice of limiting information has done more harm than good. According to these reports, patients who are not involved and informed go through many unnecessary procedures (Summers, 1985, p. 55).

The word *patient* is derived from the Latin word *patire,* to suffer. We need to keep the root of this word in mind and ask ourselves whether sometimes the agent of a patient's suffering may not be the caregiving team, as they invade, push, poke, awaken, and generally frighten the patient. One way to reduce this needless suffering is to encourage patient responsibility and involvement so that patients can provide the professional caregiver with feedback about how they are feeling and reacting to treatment.

Most health care organizations realize that patients will have to take responsibility for their own care, especially as patient stays become shorter and patients go home with a greater need for continued treatment than in the past. Successful treatment in the future will depend increasingly on the ability of patients, their families, and professionals to provide follow-up care after the hospital stay.

Patient Involvement at Planetree. Because patient involvement and shared responsibility are at the heart of patient-focused care, we will examine how these concepts are applied at Planetree. The Planetree philosophy is based on the concept that the healing process must include the patient in partnership with the professional caregivers. In order to tap the healing potential of each patient, Planetree provides a comprehensive program of patient involvement.

The focus on patient involvement begins when the patient first enters Planetree and continues throughout the patient's stay in the hospital. As soon as a patient is admitted to the Planetree unit, he meets with his physician and other members of the care team in order to discuss the treatment plan and choose the strategy that is most appropriate. In order to participate fully in these discussions, patients and their families have access to a small library on the unit and a large library across the street. Patients are also given information about their condition and recommended methods of treatment.

Unlike the staff in some institutions, the staff at Planetree encourages patients to ask questions. The staff has found that patients may be reluctant to ask questions or gather information for two reasons. Either they are afraid to know more about their condition, or they feel that they do not have the expertise to handle medical information. At Planetree, even those patients who seem not to want information or feel they are not smart enough to handle it are still encouraged to become involved.

Involvement often extends to family members, who are designated with the title "care partners." Dealing with the reactions of family members to their role as care partners has been part of a learning process for the staff at Planetree. According to Planetree's nursing coordinator, one family member was slightly intimidated by his role as care partner. This man's wife had a tracheotomy and was on a ventilator. The nursing coordinator remarked, "Although at first he reacted to the suggestion that he [might] take on some responsibility for his wife's care by bolting from the room, he became proficient at doing what needed to be done" (quoted in Jenna, 1986b, p. 54).

Another example of patient involvement is the self-medication program. Patients at Planetree are responsible for taking their own medication. Naturally, the patients are trained so that they know the dosage and the schedule. The main advantage of this program is that once patients have administered their own medication during their hospital stay, it is easy for them to continue doing so when they return home.

Another aspect of patient involvement and empowerment at Planetree is the open-chart policy. This is perhaps the most controversial aspect of the Planetree program. At Planetree patients are allowed to look at their charts and are even encouraged to write comments. When Planetree first introduced this idea, some physicians were so uncomfortable they chose not to admit patients to the unit. Others felt that knowing that patients would be looking at the chart encouraged them to write accurately and objectively. One physician observed, "The open chart policy tends to get rid of sloppy habits . . . and being aware that the patient will be reading the chart makes me think before I write. . . . It improves my chart writing" (quoted in Jenna, 1986b, p. 57). Overall, the benefits of increased patient and family involvement at Planetree include a more active role for the patient, a more satisfying relationship between patient and staff, and better care when the patient returns home.

Healing Environment

Another important aspect of patient-focused care is the creation of a healing environment, a nurturing space that can enhance the patient's healing process. The environment of the hospital can have a tremendous impact on the general well-being and attitude of patients and can influence the rate of recovery and even the amount of painkilling medicine needed.

Need for a Nurturing Environment. The following story illustrates the effect of a negative environment on a patient we will call John. John was in the hospital for a serious operation and was still in the intensive-care unit (ICU) several days after surgery. He later explained that he found the environment there so disturbing that he finally removed all the monitors and walked out. Later, a nurse found him collapsed on the floor. Following this episode he was moved out of the ICU into a regular room. Afterward he revealed that he was most disturbed by the lack of privacy and the cold, impersonal environment of the ICU.

Listen to the experience of another patient who spent four and a half weeks in the ICU. "In . . . the intensive care unit, the only window visible from my bed was across the room. Yet it was so small that I couldn't even enjoy the scenery beyond it. . . . During my first week . . . my husband brought me . . . Poinsettias. A nurse abruptly took them away explaining that plants were not allowed in the intensive care unit" (Baier, 1989, p. 14).

We may think that having a window with a view of the outside and some contact with nature is a minor consideration. However, in a study conducted at Tulane University two groups of postsurgical patients were compared over a six-year period. One group had windows in their rooms that faced a brick-walled courtyard; the other had a view of a park filled with trees, plants, and people. Comparing the rate of recovery of these two groups showed that the patients with a view of plants and the outdoors had shorter stays and took fewer painkillers than the other group (McKahan, 1991, p. 5).

It is not surprising that the latest architectural designs for hospitals take into consideration the patient's need to have contact with light, nature, and the outdoors. Modern hospital design now often includes a large atrium in the lobby with skylights to allow the maximum amount of sunlight in. In the future, perhaps all bed wings will be built around greenhouses, atriums, and courtyards. Light and nature provide an environment much more conducive to healing and the well-being of patients than the traditional windowless rooms found in many hospitals.

Another important aspect of a healing environment is the integration of food and nutrition into the healing philosophy. Although the modern hospital has no problem providing the latest treatment with the most up-to-date medical technology, it may fall short in some aspects of basic care, such as the quality of food. The following story illustrates this shortcoming.

Jane, a woman in her forties, was in the ICU of a large metropolitan hospital for six weeks and lost over twenty pounds because of the effect of the surgery and the illness itself. She was told that she had to gain weight as part of her recovery process. There was only one problem: she could not eat the "industrial" food served in the cafeteria. She finally decided to leave the hospital and go home so that she could gain her weight back. The quality of her medical care in the hospital was excellent; however, she had to leave before she could enjoy eating again.

Designing a Healing Environment at Planetree. If we begin to accept the possibility that the mind and spirit can contribute to healing, then designing supportive environments is more than a frill; it is an integral part of the healing process. For example, the Planetree unit was designed to provide a soothing, homelike environment where optimal healing can take place (Jenna, 1986a).

The most important structural additions made at Planetree were a kitchenette, where patients and their families can cook and store food, and a patient lounge for relaxing, watching videotapes, and visiting with friends and family. The designers also eliminated the traditional nursing station and replaced it with an open counter. In addition, they added many personal touches, like hand-painted ceramic tiles on the doors to indicate the room numbers. Although these changes may seem relatively minor, small details can often have the most impact on the satisfaction and well-being of patients.

At Planetree, providing nutritious and tasty food is also central to the philosophy of care. Rather than merely providing a selection of food from the hospital's kitchen, Planetree provides patients with the services of a nutritional counselor. Patients also have access to a kitchenette, which reinforces the empowerment philosophy. Patients may have a snack or cook a favorite dish whenever they would like to eat rather than being at the mercy of the institution's meal schedule.

Continuity of Care

Patient-focused care emphasizes a personalized approach by treating each individual as a unique human being rather than as a set of symptoms and classifiable diseases. This focus includes providing patients with continuity of care so that they interact with the same caregivers. Rather than seeing sixty to seventy different hospital personnel during an average six- to seven-day stay, the patient interacts with only ten caregivers. Patient satisfaction increases because patients and staff develop a close relationship. Patients feel much more comfortable seeing familiar faces rather than a parade of strangers going in and out of the room. The staff also benefits by getting to know each patient and gaining a sense of personal loyalty to and responsibility for the well-being of that patient.

Many hospitals have implemented primary nursing, in which one nurse provides most of the care for the same patient throughout the hospital stay. This form of nursing results in a strong bond between patient and nurse and also provides a comprehensive approach to patient care.

Restructuring for Decentralization

In the traditional hospital, ancillary services such as x-rays, radiology, and laboratories are located in one centralized location, which necessitates scheduling patients and transporting them to these central locations. As we shall see in Chapter Two, scheduling, coordination, and transportation often result in these procedures' taking much more time than necessary. Decentralization of ancillary services requires placing minilaboratories and x-ray facilities on the units themselves. The goal is to reduce the need for constant transportation of patients throughout the hospital and for all the voluminous paperwork and logistics that go with a highly centralized system.

Patient-focused restructuring, as this process is called, is a courageous and visionary response to both the crisis of cost and the crisis of purpose. Restructuring means that work is designed around the needs of the patient instead of the needs of specialists and departments. Restructuring a hospital's operations also means changing the nature of many caregivers' jobs and changing the environment in which they are performed. Restructuring hospital operations redirects responsibility for hospital care back to the bedside and the patient's nurse.

Elements of restructuring include streamlining supply and administrative systems, redesigning the layout of the workspace, eliminating redundant documentation and paperwork, decentralizing ancillary services, and implementing a team approach to patient care. All these elements are explored in detail in Chapter Two.

Of these elements, decentralizing ancillary services and creating a team approach to patient care have the most impact on assuring continuity of care. Decentralizing services means moving routine care functions to the patient unit. For example, the team on the unit might provide simple laboratory tests, patient transportation, routine respiratory therapy, physical therapy, admissions, electrodiagnosis, and a host of other procedures. Also a satellite pharmacy or laboratory module might be relocated to the unit. These changes help to integrate personnel into a single team focused on providing timely services to customers. In this model, caregivers perform most of the tasks previously performed by a variety of departments, each with its own highly specialized role.

Cross-Training and Multiskilled Practitioners

Patient-focused care changes the emphasis from having specialized staff with narrow role definitions to cross-training staff so they become multiskilled practitioners. Cross-training goes hand in hand with restructuring. Ideally, caregivers are drawn from a variety of backgrounds related to the patient population's needs. For example, an orthopedic unit may develop teams with physical therapists and radiology technicians who, in turn, are trained to do basic patient-care activities. They may provide care in partnership with a professional nurse, who is also cross-trained. After training, these practitioners are prepared to do respiratory therapy, electrocardigrams, scheduling, charting at bedside computers, medical records, and a variety of other activities that do not fit traditional job descriptions. With this model, caregivers are rewarded for flexibility through a range of pay scales.

In one hospital that has restructured its operations, teams of two caregivers, known as "care pairs," shoulder the full range of direct patient-care responsibilities from admitting and charting to transportation and from room cleanup to care planning, assessment, and therapeutic intervention (Weber, 1991, p. 25).

Multiskilled practitioners can be organized in teams of two or three that provide care for three to five patients throughout their hospital stay. This practice results in continuity of care as patients interact with only a few caregivers and have the opportunity to form relationships with them.

Holistic Approach

Another important aspect of patient-focused care is the holistic approach, which integrates the mind, body, and spirit in the healing process. The underlying assumption of the holistic model of medicine is that treating any illness must go beyond merely addressing the symptoms of the specific disease to take into account the underlying causes of the condition.

The holistic approach includes a variety of techniques and treatments, but the basic premise is that any disorder in any part of the person is a signal that an imbalance exists in the entire mind/body system. Symptoms are merely the surface manifestations of a basic disharmony at deeper levels of being. As a result, disease is seen as a process rather than as a thing. Any attempts at treatment, therefore, must address the whole person and take into account the role of the mind, belief systems, and thoughts in the genesis of illness.

In the allopathic model of medicine, body and mind are seen as separate systems. This view leads to a separation of treatment approaches so that one kind of practitioner handles mental/emotional disturbances and other types of physicians handle all other illnesses. In this medical model, the mind is believed to have a secondary role or none at all in causing organic illnesses. This assumption leads to certain conclusions about prevention and treatment. The placebo effect, for example, is explained as evidence of the power of suggestion rather than as evidence of the mind's active role both in causing disease and in contributing to healing. With this model, disease prevention is based on environmental factors and emphasizes such tactics as exercising, taking vitamins, and not smoking. Although all these strategies are indeed important for preventing disease, one can also perhaps use proactive approaches to harness the power of the mind to affect the body.

Although some of the mind/body therapies available to today's health care consumer are beginning to gain acceptance by the medical establishment, many are greeted with suspicion or dismissed. Widespread prejudice still exists against forms of treatment that do not fit into the existing paradigm of Western medicine, despite evidence that some of these strategies produce measurable results.

The power of the mind to alleviate pain, prevent illness, and contribute to the healing process has hardly been tapped by modern medical practice. An article in *Time* magazine, "Why New Age Medicine Is Catching On" (Wallis, 1991, p. 68), provides evidence of the increasing availability and acceptance of alternative therapies. According to this article, these therapies are gaining in popularity because American consumers are beginning to realize that there are certain limitations to traditional medicine, and many are willing to try other approaches when the traditional approach does not work.

According to this article, conventional medicine is most successful in crisis intervention: in fixing a sprain or break, in attacking fevers, and in treating disease by the use of surgery and drugs. Traditional medicine has been far less successful in preventing, curing, or even treating chronic diseases such as lower-back pain, high blood pressure, some forms of cancer, and coronary-artery disease.

The health care industry needs to pay attention to the fact that American consumers are willing to accept alternative approaches to healing. If the medical establishment is not willing to embrace these new therapies, consumers can easily take their business elsewhere. According to Dr. Depak Chopra, a Massachusetts physician quoted in the *Time* article, the baby-boomer generation wants more than traditional medicine can offer. Furthermore, they are open-minded enough to experiment with these alternative approaches, especially when they are dissatisfied with traditional approaches that do not seem to be succeeding (p. 69).

Some of the mind/body therapies that we will explore in this book are various relaxation techniques, visualization and imagery, therapeutic touch, and counseling.

Streamlining Documentation

One of the systems that needs to be streamlined in the hospital is the amount of documentation. In the average hospital, documentation and recordkeeping occupy much more time than is necessary. Inch-thick medical records are not unusual for an average hospital stay.

One of the solutions to this problem is to reduce charting time by making documentation protocol-driven and exception-based. In other words, only exceptions to normal recovery and care are noted on the patient's chart and record. In this model, a check mark indicates that the patient's condition is within normal limits. In order to speed up the notation process medical signs that relate to cognitive, cardiovascular, pulmonary, and digestive functions can be codified and then easily recorded on the patient record. Because studies have shown that a nurse may spend up to 30 percent of his time on documentation, much of it on recordkeeping and charting, this system has the potential to greatly increase the satisfaction of nursing staff and increase the time spent in direct patient care.

All these elements are part of the patient-focused hospital. Patient-focused restructuring is indeed a revolutionary new model if one considers that it runs counter to the traditional organizational structure of the hospital. It runs counter to policies and procedures, to the way health care workers were educated and trained, to the way we promote and reward.

The difference between the provider-focused and the patient-focused approach is profound: an understanding that hospital services and medical practices must revolve around patient needs instead of personal or departmental needs. Health care practitioners cannot afford to ignore the concept of the patient at the center. Patients are becoming increasingly knowledgeable about and are demanding quality service.

"Few will challenge the goals of the patient-focused hospital. Many will question the means — telling us 'you can't get there from here.' The simple imperative is: We must get there, and here is the only place we can start. As long as we keep patients and common sense foremost in our minds, we will succeed" (Lathrop, 1991, p. 20).

The transition to a patient-focused model is neither simple nor quick, and it requires vision, commitment, and raw courage — a willingness to swim against the prevailing current. Perhaps what is now seen as experimental will one day become the norm for all hospitals. In this way, the hospital of today will become the healing center of the future.

In this chapter we have begun our exploration of the elements of patient-focused care. The rest of this book will explore these concepts in detail.

Chapter 2

The Bottom Lines: Reducing Costs and Improving Quality

First, you have to understand what a hospital is. It is a
business organization . . . which sells certain tests, remedies,
and procedures related to disease. Because the staff stays in the
hospital and the patients come and go, they eventually begin
more and more to see the hospital procedures as something
that should be designed for their own comfort and convenience,
rather than the patients'.

Lawrence LeShan,
*Cancer as a Turning Point**

Designing hospital procedures for the comfort of staff and
to follow tradition is not viable in an age of spiraling health care
costs, managed care, and the DRG system. The traditional hospital was designed to respond to cost-based reimbursement and
the special interests of health care professionals. Once a centralized structure with its emphasis on professional specialization
was in place, this way of delivering patient care became the norm.

This structure was characterized by centralized ancillary
services and all the coordination and scheduling needed to maintain this system; highly specialized roles for nursing staff and
technicians; and enormous amounts of documentation. This way
of operating may have worked in the days of cost-based reimbursement, when physicians and hospitals could set prices for
services and expect to be paid accordingly by insurers and third-

*Lawrence LeShan, *Cancer as a Turning Point,* © 1989 by Lawrence
LeShan, Ph.D. Used by permission of the publisher, Dutton, an imprint of New
American Library, a division of Penguin Books USA Inc.

27

party payers; however, it cannot work in today's environment. In the past, the high costs of inefficiency were absorbed by those who paid for the services. There was no incentive to examine operations for possible inefficiencies, and there was no pressure to cut costs.

Under a capitation system such a hospital is paid a predetermined amount regardless of the cost of the care. A hospital must be able to deliver at or below the established cost or suffer the consequences of decreased profitability. Hospitals can no longer afford inefficiency and poor-quality service because inefficiency, poor productivity, and incorrect use of resources affect their long-term success. Therefore, the emphasis under the DRG system must be to hold costs down by increasing efficiency and reducing wasted resources and duplication of services. In addition, under systems such as managed care and DRG, enhancing healing through education and high-touch therapies has important economic benefits because hospital stays are shortened. As one hospital director remarked when he first had to confront the effects of the DRG system on the hospital's budget and operating expenses: "Within the month we had to cut costs by a million and a half dollars. Our focus tightened and we became concerned with getting people out of the hospital much sooner" (quoted in Zemke, 1987, p. 41).

The DRG system is not the only reason hospitals need to be concerned about being cost effective. If hospitals are not efficiently run and if they cannot keep costs at a reasonable level, payers, such as insurance companies and employers, will simply take their business to competing hospitals. One of the new forms of managed care is employer-provided partnerships, in which the hospital and a specific employer form a partnership for taking care of the health needs of employees working for that company. If such arrangements become popular, hospitals will have to be able to compete to win clients. The strategies that hospitals can use to achieve this competitive advantage include implementing effective patient-care management systems, being dedicated to enhancing health promotion and prevention, and having a customer-oriented culture (Pavia and Berry, 1991, p. 24). All these elements will be explored in this chapter, which examines the restructuring of hospital operations in order to decentralize services.

The challenge for any hospital administrator is to reduce costs and inefficiency while, at the same time, increasing quality and offering excellent customer service. Unfortunately, the traditional structure of hospitals often prevents the achievement of these goals because of the built-in inefficiencies of the system. Patient-focused restructuring has provided some dramatic solutions to these problems. It aims to reduce waste and inefficiency, to improve quality of services, and to increase profitability.

This chapter outlines the impressive improvements resulting from implementing patient-focused restructuring. Before examining this concept closely, we need to explore the inefficiencies built into the traditional structure of hospital operations. However, we must keep in mind that it is still too early to tell conclusively how patient-focused restructuring efforts will translate into specific savings. We need more time and we need to collect more data from organizations that are currently involved with this process.

Inefficiency and Waste

The hospitals that we will be examining in this chapter have undertaken patient-focused restructuring efforts in order to increase efficiency, to improve service, and to reduce costs. They all began by utilizing the services of consulting firms that specialize in analyzing hospital operations to pinpoint opportunities for increasing efficiency.

Results of Research

On the basis of more than three years of this type of research, these firms have concluded that the primary cause of high costs, inefficiency, and poor service is the large amount of compartmentalization and specialization in today's hospital. Specialization results in hospital personnel who can perform only their own narrow duties even if they spend much of their time being idle while waiting for the next patient. Specialization also means that many separate job classifications exist in one hospital. For example, one hospital reported four different classifications for four housekeepers who clean different types of flooring. One consultant explained it this way: hospitals operate with "lots and lots of . . . small, clinically focused nursing units—almost always with dedicated staff. These multiple compartments are augmented by a baroque array of centrally dispatched phlebotomists and technicians" (Lathrop, 1991, p. 19). As a result of the built-in inefficiency of this approach, simple processes such as electrocardiograms (EKGs) can become "nightmares of coordination" with 75 percent of total personnel costs accounted for by infrastructure and structured idle time (p. 19). The overall conclusion of these studies is that improvement does not lie in making people work harder; it lies in changing the structure of hospital operations.

Another contributing factor to inefficient operations is the "application of the concept of the highest common denominator" (Lathrop, 1991, p. 19). In other words, procedures are designed to handle the most acute cases: patients with extremely complex medical needs. This approach breeds waste and poor management because only a small percentage of patients fall into the highest-common-denominator category. Sixty to 80 percent of patient care is routine. Another problem with designing hospital operations around the needs of the most acute cases is that the system then depends on "exploiting differences, not [on] forcing similarities" (p. 19). By designing services around the needs of the sickest patients, we lose the leverage needed to cut costs and provide prompt, efficient service.

As a result of the inefficiencies built into the system, turnaround times for tests are much longer than they have to be, continuity of care is rare, and costs for coordinating and scheduling services are much higher than necessary. Specific examples of waste and inefficiency are provided by hospitals that have restructured services.

Bishop Clarkson. Bishop Clarkson Memorial Hospital in Omaha found that documentation consumed more time than actual patient care. (All information about Bishop Clarkson in this chapter comes from Anthony, 1991.) Documentation accounted for 29 percent of one unit's total work hours, while medical, technical, and clinical tasks consumed only 16 percent of the staff's time. The average employee was idle for about ninety minutes, or 18 percent of each eight-hour working day, while 12 percent of the day (one hour) was set aside for scheduling and coordinating. Clarkson also learned that respiratory therapists were able to administer care during only one-half of their visits to patients because often the therapist did not know that the nurse had scheduled other procedures for that time.

Redundancy was another factor contributing to inefficiency. Clarkson found that patients sometimes had their vital signs taken four times in fifteen minutes because each of the four clinicians who had treated these patients were required to perform this task as part of their routine.

Clarkson also found unnecessary complexity in performing such routine procedures as taking x-rays. A typical x-ray, for example, took ninety minutes and involved forty-seven steps, even though the procedure itself took only ten minutes. The rest of the time was lost in scheduling, transportation, and documentation.

Lakeland Regional Medical Center. Lakeland Regional Medical Center in Florida, another hospital that underwent an operational analysis of its structure, discovered a high degree of compartmentalization and complexity. (Unless otherwise noted, all information about Lakeland in this chapter comes from Weber, 1991.) For example, the medical center had 400 job descriptions in seventy different departments. As Dr. David Jones, the medical director at Lakeland, remarked, "When you think about that number, it's incredible. . . . We've made things so complex" (quoted in Loudin, 1991, p. 4).

Lakeland found a similar level of complexity as Clarkson in the performance of routine services. An x-ray, for example, involved fifteen to twenty employees, required forty steps, and took 140 minutes; it required only six of these steps and 20 minutes to take the x-ray (Loudin, 1991, p. 4). The rest of the time was spent waiting, coordinating, and scheduling.

Lakeland also found that a nurse's time was not used productively. Nurses spent 29 percent of their precious time and energy scribbling down observations including such remarks as "skin warm and dry. . . . Patient slept well." They also found that documenting assessments and care plans took more time than actual assessment and caregiving. Inch-thick medical records for an average stay in the hospital were not at all unusual.

Other Hospitals. Other hospitals found similar evidence of complexity and specialization. St. Vincent in Indianapolis found that it had 598 job classifications with six associates per class. Lee Memorial Medical Center in Fort Myers, Florida, found that it had 437 job classifications and six to eight layers of management. Lee Memorial also found that one stroke victim could interact with as many as 105 hospital personnel during a six-day stay. (Unless otherwise noted, all information in this chapter about St. Vincent and Lee Memorial comes from Weber, 1991.)

To summarize, many of the hospitals that underwent operational analysis by consultants came to the following conclusions (Chicago Health Executives Forum, 1991, p. 12):

> Work is fragmented, process intensive, and compartmentalized.
> Time is wasted by caregivers' waiting, coordinating, and scheduling.
> Administrative barriers block efficiency.
> Continuity and quality of care is low due to the large number of caregivers involved in caring for one patient.
> Duplication occurs between departments.
> Hospital operations and policies are driven by the needs of departments rather than the needs of patients.

Costs of Inefficiency

All these examples of inefficiency and waste affect the bottom line, especially if they result in idle time and duplication of effort. For every dollar spent on direct care, hospitals spend three to four dollars waiting for it to happen, preparing to do it, and writing it down. "Recording, scheduling, transporting, supervising, attending meetings, tidying up, serving meals, and standing around consume 84 percent of personnel activities" (Weber, 1991, p. 24).

Patient-focused restructuring addresses these issues by cutting down on labor costs through decentralizing ancillary services and cross-training personnel to be able to perform several jobs. These changes reduce coordination and scheduling time and also decrease idle time for all personnel. Because wages, salaries, and benefits constitute more than one-half of a typical hospital's costs, a reduction in personnel can allow the hospital to invest in other things such as new equipment. "If you can send $10,000 worth of labor out the door, . . . you can afford to buy $75,000 or $100,000 worth of equipment" (Weber, 1991, p. 24).

One need only examine the figures below to realize how wasteful and inefficient the system is (Lathrop, 1991, p. 181).

> Fourteen cents out of every dollar spent on wages is consumed trying to schedule and coordinate medical care.
> Twenty-nine cents of every wage dollar goes for documentation (most of it done by nurses).
> Twenty cents of the wage dollar pays for structured idle time.
> Thirty-seven cents of the wage dollar goes for everything else—hotel and patient services, transportation, management, and supervision.

Looking for Solutions: Restructuring Hospital Operation₃

What is the solution? The solution does not lie in working harder and faster. Most cost-reduction strategies in the past have focused on having people work faster; however, this solution does not begin to address the root of the problem. "Once you've decided you are going to have centralized phlebotomy, you've dealt the hand. . . . It doesn't matter how fast the poor phlebotomist runs from room to room" (Weber, 1991, p. 24). The answer lies in altering the structure of hospital operations, for changing the structure promotes real productivity and quality (Weber, 1991, p. 19).

The goal of patient-focused restructuring is to increase the amount of time that caregivers can spend in direct care, to improve the quality of care, and, at the same time, to lower personnel-related costs. Although the elimination of waste and duplication is the primary goal, another equally important benefit of this process is creating high-quality customer service, an efficient place to work, and a humane, caring environment for patients.

Patient-focused restructuring decreases the amount of time spent in scheduling, coordinating, and documentation, thereby giving caregivers more time to spend with patients. As a result, staff members are more satisfied because they spend time in direct patient care rather than on clerical tasks. This point is crucial because the only way to excel in a service industry is by having a motivated, committed workforce involved in jobs that they enjoy doing.

Restructuring also allows staff time for patient support and education, which has been proven to shorten the length of hospital stays by decreasing complications, improving respiratory function, and decreasing psychological distress. In an analysis of 191 studies, the effects of psychoeducational interventions for surgical patients decreased the length of stay by an average of 1.5 days (12 percent) (Sobel, 1992).

Reasons for Restructuring

Before examining the major elements of patient-focused restructuring, we will outline the characteristics of several hospitals across the country that have embarked on major restructuring programs and examine their reasons for doing so. The hospitals that we will examine are Bishop Clarkson Memorial Hospital in Omaha, Nebraska; Lee Memorial Hospital in Fort Myers, Florida; Lakeland Regional Medical Center in Lakeland, Florida; St. Vincent Hospital and Healthcare Center in Indianapolis; and Vanderbilt University Medical Center in Nashville.

All these hospitals are large, not-for-profit institutions and have 300 to over 500 beds. All are short-term, acute-care facilities. All had a strong financial position before beginning the patient-focused project; however, they had concerns about maintaining financial stability in the future. They wanted to improve operational effectiveness and quality of care in order to strengthen their competitive position and increase their appeal to customers (Chicago Health Executives Forum, 1991, p. 11).

These institutions decided to implement restructuring efforts in order to attempt to meet the challenges they were facing. These challenges included personnel shortages, recruitment and retention problems, reduced reimbursements, increased competition, a decrease in census, and, on the positive side, a drive to be customer-focused and to respond to patient needs. Although most health care providers face similar challenges, these hospitals had the driving force of a visionary chief executive officer (CEO) and an executive team willing to take the risks involved in embarking on this change process.

Most of these hospitals utilized the expertise of consultants to assist in this process. Some hospitals are presently working on restructuring their operations with only minimal help from outside consultants. Usually, these hospitals use consultants only to initiate the process. There is one important consideration in deciding whether to use outside consultants. A consulting firm has the advantage of being entirely objective about the information they find as they conduct their analysis. They have no vested interest in having the data look more positive than it actually is. Therefore, it may be helpful to employ outside consultants not just for their expertise but because of their objectivity and ability to evaluate results without prejudice.

Evaluating Readiness for Change

Successful restructuring efforts depend on a careful assessment of the unique characteristics and requirements of the organization. There is no one-size-fits-all model that will work with all hospitals. Each hospital needs to assess its current status and examine options for future development. Among the factors that need to be considered are current operating capability and efficiency and the ability of the organization to create a culture that supports change.

A framework that can be used to analyze an organization's readiness for restructuring is a continuum of organizational and operational development. This continuum, developed by a group of consultants, contains four stages (Allawi, Bellaire, and David, 1991, p. 39). The hospitals that we will be examining in this chapter were all at a fairly high level of development on this continuum; however, hospitals in the future that will be undertaking restructuring efforts will probably include some that are in financial trouble and facing other significant problems.

A hospital at the *first stage* of development, called the "survival" stage, needs to change because it is losing money: it is either in default already or is operating with a negative profit margin. Often, change is blocked by scarce resources and lack of ability. A hospital at the survival stage may also not have efficiently functioning basic systems, characterized by high error rates in such processes as patient admissions. The goal of the restructuring process of a hospital in the survival stage is to develop standards and systems for managing operations as well as new management tools.

A hospital in the *second stage,* known as the "defense" stage, is usually in a stronger organizational position than a hospital in the first stage. It usually has a strong management system and an acceptable financial position. Its primary challenge is to prepare for future competitive challenges by focusing on ways to differentiate itself from the competition. The goal is to pinpoint areas where the hospital can gain a leadership position.

The hospital in the *third stage,* known as the "differentiation" stage, is profitable and a market leader with ample resources to maintain that position and to make changes. The challenge is to maintain success. The goal is to develop specific products that will differentiate it from the competition and place it in a "world-class" position. Such a hospital still cannot afford to count on past successes; it must continually strive to outdo itself in order to remain competitive.

The *fourth stage,* the "domination" position, is an ideal that hospitals are striving toward but that none has yet achieved. In this stage, the organization is characterized by flexibility in responding to changes in customer needs in order to remain competitive. Such a hospital would be dedicated to remaining at the cutting edge of the industry; it would have a highly service-oriented culture and multiple product lines at optimal levels, and would provide the best outcomes at the lowest possible cost.

As will become evident as we study examples of hospitals that have restructured, restructuring requires establishing a culture that supports the dramatic changes that will occur not only in operations but also in job design and management structure. An organization undergoing the restructuring process needs to provide direction and support for all personnel and needs to seek input and participation from all levels of the organization during this change process.

It is important to gain support and commitment for the vision and goals of the patient-focused philosophy. Commitment, active participation, and support from top management are essential in any process like this because it requires a major shift in organizational culture and values. Top management needs to provide training for all staff in team building, decision making, communication skills, and problem solving.

Although patient-focused restructuring has produced dramatic results in patient and staff satisfaction, all staff will not automatically embrace the changes that occur as a result of this process. Some employees will be uncomfortable with their new roles and increased autonomy, so some turnover may be inevitable. The ongoing need for training and team building will require investment of both time and energy.

Planning for Restructuring

After a thorough analysis as outlined here, hospitals should implement patient-focused restructuring only after extensive planning. Trends in service needs must be considered. For example, whether a specific service will continue to be an inpatient service or whether it will become available on an outpatient basis must be considered before making any decisions about restructuring. Decentralization requires a certain amount of patient homogeneity and is dependent on a specific volume on a unit; therefore, decentralization should not be planned when the population is heterogeneous or when the volume does not justify the effort based on a careful cost-benefit analysis (Chicago Health Executives Forum, 1991, p. 30).

Hospitals that conclude that complete reorganization is not feasible can implement some of the elements of the patient-focused model. For example, some hospitals are implementing the cross-training of staff in order to better utilize patient-care staff. For hospitals considering this approach, it is crucial to analyze the volume of ancillary services. Also, regulatory guidelines must be taken into account.

Another element of patient-focused restructuring that can be implemented on its own is charting-by-exception and the development of patient-care protocols. Bedside computer terminals are an important aid for this process.

Patient-focused restructuring should not be undertaken with the illusion that the institution will see a dramatic decrease in cost or a quick gain in market share. These results may occur in the long run; however, they should not be expected in the short run.

Elements of Restructuring

The patient-focused concept is based on the belief that quality and profit can be improved by restructuring organizations. The elements of this innovative approach to patient-care delivery are discussed in this section.

Decentralization of Services

The goal of decentralization is to move clinical, administrative, and ancillary services close to the patient rather than transporting patients to centralized departments in other areas of the hospital. Transporting patients for laboratory work, x-rays, and other diagnostic procedures is both inefficient and time-consuming. Decentralization saves time and coordination by bringing these services to the patient.

According to the results of operational-analysis studies, the high personnel costs associated with ancillary services is due to the amount of scheduling, coordination, documentation, and transportation needed to perform these services. The goal of having unit-based ancillary services is to be able to perform most routine procedures right on the unit, thereby eliminating the need for patients to be transported all over the hospital and reducing the number of caregivers that patients interact with.

For example, Lakeland Regional Medical Center turned a forty-bed unit into a self-contained surgical service with its own minilab, diagnostic rooms, supply stockroom, and administrative records/clinical area. At Bishop Clarkson Memorial Hospital, ancillary services, including administrative, laboratory, and radiology services, were decentralized and moved to the same floor as patient rooms. The goal is to be able to meet 90 percent of the pre- and postsurgical needs of patients on the unit. Patient servers house supplies, including medication, charts, linen, and dressings. Bedside computer terminals aid in documentation, ancillary-service scheduling, and ordering supplies.

The decision as to what type of ancillary services to decentralize depends on the patient population and the kind of services they need. Most patient-focused units are larger than traditional units. For example, a traditional unit may have twenty-five to thirty beds, while a patient-focused unit may have forty to eighty beds.

Cross-Training

The goal of cross-training is to eliminate specialization and decrease the number of caregivers who interact with patients. On patient-focused units, caregivers are cross-trained to meet 80 percent to 90 percent of a patient's needs including x-rays, routine laboratory work, EKGs, traditional nursing, and respiratory care. Caregivers from a variety of backgrounds are cross-trained. As outlined in Chapter Three, there are many models for setting up teams of multi-skilled practitioners.

At Lakeland, for example, teams are made up of a care pair, usually a registered nurse and a cross-trained technician. Each care pair on each shift can meet up to 90 percent of the pre- and postsurgical needs of four to seven patients. Each care pair at Lakeland is backed by a unit-based pharmacist, a unit clerk, and a unit support aide to help with transportation, supply restocking, upkeep, and maintenance.

At Lakeland, cross-training is provided for nurses (LVNs and LPNs), patient-care assistants (PCAs), respiratory therapists, and radiological technicians. Training for the pilot project included six weeks of full-time classes followed by competency-based testing in the following areas: phlebotomy, EKG, respiratory and physical therapy, laboratory testing, and diagnostic radiology procedures. The goal is for the care pairs to be able to handle all patient care, hotel functions, and records processing. Their motto is "never pass over something you can do yourself . . . and . . . do more and more things for fewer people."

The results of patient-focused care at Lakeland include a 9.2 percent savings on direct bedside-care costs, from $13,256 in a traditional unit to $12,034 in the patient-focused unit. Another important benefit is that the care pairs double the amount of time available for direct patient care, from 21 percent to 53 percent of total time.

At Clarkson, cross-training is based on care partnerships consisting of a pair of care providers. The pair consists of a registered nurse and a partner who could be a respiatory therapist, medical technician, or x-ray technician. Each partnership has responsibility for six to twelve patients. St. Vincent in Indianapolis uses care trios, a cross-trained RN working with two other cross-trained, technically skilled personnel.

At Vanderbilt University Medical Center in Nashville, three classes of multiskilled personnel — clinical associates, administrative assistants, and service associates — work collaboratively. For example, administrative assistants are trained to do admitting, insurance verification, coding, and completion of medical records, in addition to unit reception and hotel services. In order to reduce the time for cross-training at Vanderbilt, the decision was made to limit the skills to those that one "needs to know" rather than to include those that are "nice to know." (All information about Vanderbilt in this chapter comes from Weber, 1991.) Training on the patient-focused units concentrates on both clinical skills and interpersonal skills such as group dynamics, team building, negotiating, and communication. Some pilot units are cross-training radiological technicians to perform bedside nursing tasks in order to utilize their time efficiently when they are not doing x-rays for the unit's patients. Other patient-focused care units have cross-trained RNs to perform some laboratory work.

One of the obstacles to extensive cross-training may be

allied health licensing regulations, which may not allow certain professions or technicians to perform some functions. Some state professional-practice acts prevent hospitals from cross-training in any of another professional's skills. For example, in Indiana, radiology work can be done only by licensed radiology technicians. In Tennessee, laboratory activities cannot be performed by anyone other than a certified laboratory technician (Chicago Health Executives Forum, 1991, p. 17).

Cross-training solves one of the major inefficiencies of the traditional hospital structure: idle time. In the patient-focused model, laboratory technicians not only perform blood tests and other laboratory tasks but are also cross-trained to help with drawing blood, to transport patients, and to assist nurses in moving patients. These tasks fill in what would otherwise be unused portions of the day and can also make the job interesting. One benefit of cross-training is that the number of vacant positions can be decreased by filling them with cross-trained staff. This flexibility is especially crucial for institutions that have significant shortages of professional staff.

Continuity of Care

One of the goals of patient-focused restructuring is to provide continuity of care. In this model, caregivers truly "own" their patient because continuity can be maintained across shifts and across days. Three-day-stay patients no longer interact with fifty-five employees; they may interact with fewer than fifteen. For example, at Lee Memorial Medical Center each patient is the responsibility of a case coordinator from the time of admission to the time of discharge. At Robert Wood Johnson University Hospital in New Brunswick, New Jersey, management and coordination of individual patient care are done by an RN clinical-care manager who is responsible for about a dozen patients. (All information about Robert Wood Johnson in this chapter comes from Weber, 1991.)

At Lakeland with its care pairs, continuity of care is maintained because these pairs fulfill most of the needs of four to seven patients. Patients interact only with their own team of caregivers. Compared with traditional nursing service, care pairs can double the amount of time they spend catering to a patient's medical, technical, and clinical needs. On the patient-focused unit at Lakeland, nurses spend 53 percent of the day in direct patient contact, while on the other units nurses spend only 21 percent of their day in direct patient care. On the patient-focused unit, a patient interacts with thirteen hospital personnel during an average stay in the hospital. This is 75 percent fewer than the twenty-seven nurses, ten dietary personnel, six ancillary-services personnel, five transportation personnel, and three environmental-services personnel who interact with one patient during an average stay on other units (Weber, 1991, p. 25). Continuity of care extends to physicians. More than 60 percent of patients on the patient-focused unit are seen exclusively by their primary physician throughout their hospitalization.

Redesigning the Workspace

Because patient-focused restructuring involves streamlining supply and administrative systems and decentralizing ancillary services, it is obvious that the physical workplace needs to be redesigned. Renovating existing space or designing new space must be done in ways that embrace the patient-centered philosophy.

At Bishop Clarkson Memorial Hospital, for example, patient servers replaced the nursing station's previous storage functions. Patient servers were built directly into every room to provide storage for supplies, some drugs, and commonly used items such as bandages, syringes, tubing, patient records, and nursing notes.

The patient-focused unit at Clarkson also has bedside computer terminals to assist in documentation, ancillary-service scheduling, and ordering of supplies. The terminals were initially used mainly for supply ordering. They are now being used to order laboratory tests, to schedule EKGs, and to document physicians' orders. Supplies are ordered by sweeping the scanner across the bar code printed on the supply packaging. The patient's chart, care documentation, and physician's orders, all of which used to be stored at the nursing station, are now stored in patient rooms. These computers can also be used for obtaining reports from pathology and from radiology. The unit was also refitted with a satellite x-ray unit and a satellite laboratory. The cost for remodeling the fifty-one-bed patient-focused unit was $1.3 million — $700,000 for physical renovation and $600,000 for new x-ray and laboratory equipment.

The Planetree unit provides another example of workplace redesigning. The idea was to transform a typical hospital environment into a comfortable, homelike environment. One of the first changes was to redesign the existing nurse station into an open and airy workspace by removing the standard partition between patients and staff. The physical environment reinforces egalitarian interaction, a concept that is central to Planetree. Other changes included adding wood surfaces to replace the institutional look of stainless steel and changing to a softer form of lighting. Ceramic tiles were used to designate room numbers (Jenna, 1986b).

Reducing Documentation

Because one of the goals of the patient-focused unit is to reduce unnecessary paperwork and decrease documentation, all models of patient-focused care have adopted some way of streamlining medical records. Charting-by-exception is based on documenting a patient's medical signs only when there is a significant change from the norm. With this method, protocols of care need to be developed. These protocols define for a given diagnosis the plan of care for medical, nursing, and ancillary procedures by day of stay. Although these protocols are applicable to some patients, such as surgical or orthopedic patients or others with homogeneous diagnoses, they may not work as well with patients who have several clinical issues and therefore may not lend themselves to predictable pathways of care.

This procedure can dramatically reduce the time nurses spend in documentation from 29 percent to a mere 2 percent of the typical day. At Lee Memorial, for example, the implementation of this simplified system resulted in a net savings of forty-three minutes per caregiver shift.

Management of Units

The management of a patient-focused unit is different from the management of a traditional nursing unit. Patient-focused units are usually managed by a unit manager, who may or may not be an RN. The role of this unit manager is different from the traditional role of the head nurse. Unit managers have to maintain a "dotted-line" relationship with central departments. The unit manager has to have knowledge of all ancillary functions because all personnel, including both ancillary-service and nursing personnel, report to this manager. In sharp contrast, a head nurse has responsibility for nursing personnel but no authority over ancillary departments.

In several patient-focused hospitals, the goal is to further flatten the management structure by having the care teams do evaluation, supervision, and problem resolution. Under a model called shared leadership, decision making is decentralized so that staff has responsibility for decisions that affect cost and quality (Lathrop, 1991, p. 19).

Results of Restructuring

According to one CEO, the benefits of patient-focused care include significant quality improvements and "increased customer satisfaction which can translate into increased market share, decreased patient length-of-stay, personnel retention benefits and labor cost reductions adding up to 7% of operating expense" (Weber, 1991, p. 30).

According to results at Robert Wood Johnson University Hospital, benefits include improved quality of care and increased employee and patient satisfaction. One of the dramatic effects on the bottom line has been a 26 percent reduction in length of stay, which has allowed the hospital to admit more patients. For example, according to Mary Tonges, vice-president of nursing at Johnson, the new system could generate as much as 105 extra admissions annually in surgical orthopedics—an estimated $700,000 in additional revenue.

Despite some risks and the need for further analysis to

determine the financial and quality-improvement advantages of patient-focused care, this model has already shown some dramatic results. We will now examine specific results in several areas.

Increased Physician and Staff Satisfaction

Patient-focused restructuring results in measurable improvement in satisfaction for physicians and other staff. At Lakeland, the care-pair model has doubled the amount of time that caregivers spend with patients, from 21 percent of the day to 53 percent. Time spent with patients has had a positive effect on staff satisfaction levels, especially among nurses.

Nursing Turnover. Typically, nursing turnover in a hospital's patient-focused-care unit is the lowest of any of the units. Lower turnover has a significant cost benefit because it costs $1,000, on average, to orient a new nurse. Clarkson indicated that nurse satisfaction increased from 50 percent to 70 percent with patient-focused care. Nurses are especially pleased with the patient-focused-care unit because it allows them to spend more time on actual bedside care. At St. Vincent, in the past nurses spent only 46 percent of their time at the patient's bedside; now, they can spend 65 percent. Bedside hours per patient day rose from 6.2 to 8 as a result of restructuring. Lakeland reported a lower RN turnover rate on the patient-focused unit. One of the important contributing factors to increased nurse satisfaction is the fact that nurses have more input regarding patient care on the patient-focused unit than on other units. As one care partner at Clarkson mentioned, "You don't have to rush to complete your work. . . . You have much more control over the whole flow of your patient's day."

Physician Satisfaction. Physicians report increased satisfaction based on significant improvement in nursing care and in the quality of test results, reduced turnaround time, reduced paperwork, and increased efficiency. At Lee Memorial, physician survey results were more positive in five or six categories than results for the rest of the hospital. Physicians generally were pleased and felt that continuity of care was better on the patient-focused units than with the traditional delivery systems. The only area of concern for physicians was communication because physician rounds were no longer conducted in the traditional manner.

At St. Vincent, a survey revealed that on the conventional unit, 64 percent of physicians were satisfied with the service; however, only 14 percent reported that they were "very satisfied." On the patient-focused unit, 65 percent reported they were "very satisfied" and 35 percent reported overall satisfaction (Weber, 1991, p. 26). As far as meeting the physicians' immediate needs, 90 percent of the physicians were "very satisfied" with the patient-focused unit as compared with only 62 percent reporting high levels of satisfaction previously.

Employee Satisfaction. Most patient-focused units also reported an increase in employee satisfaction. Employees found that patient-focused care improved their work environment. As one employee at Clarkson commented, "You have more control over the situation between yourself and the patient." At Lakeland, an employee evaluation survey indicated that job stress decreased on the patient-focused unit. At Vanderbilt University Medical Center, 80 percent of the staff on the patient-focused unit were satisfied with the documentation requirements; employees on a traditional unit expressed 0 percent satisfaction. At Lee Memorial, employees stated that they would not want to return to a traditional-care delivery system. At St. Vincent, staff reported a sense of belonging to a team and increased control over patient care (Chicago Health Executives Forum, 1991, p. 22). Clarkson found that staff working in the patient-focused unit was one-third less likely than staff on other units to say that the work load hindered quality. There was also a 50 percent reduction in negative feedback about the physical layout and how that affected the staff's ability to respond to patient needs.

Recruitment and Retention. However, there are mixed reviews regarding the effect of patient-focused restructuring on the recruitment and retention of staff. Because patient-focused care involves a tremendous change process, the amount of change may directly affect retention and recruitment patterns. One of the concerns is that ancillary-personnel turnover rates may increase because of the blurring of professional and nonprofessional roles in the patient-focused unit. Another concern is that staff who are part of the change process may be worried about job security.

Increased Patient Satisfaction. During this time of intense competition and in an era dedicated to quality improvement and service excellence, improving patient satisfaction is a major goal for all hospitals. Clarkson found that in the patient-focused units patient perceptions of nursing care, hospital environment, and concern for the patient rose from the thirteenth to the ninety-second percentile in Gallup-SRI patient satisfaction surveys. This is certainly a significant difference. At the same time, length of stay decreased by 10 percent. Satisfaction levels were 13 percent to 17 percent higher on these units than on conventional units.

The patient-focused unit at St. Vincent received a much higher rating on room cleanliness: 86 percent versus only 77 percent on other units. Patients also commented on prompt call-light response, clear instructions, prompt solution of problems, and good staff teamwork. On this unit, 90 percent of patients said that nurses showed concern for them as individuals, compared with 77 percent on the other units. At Lee Memorial, patient surveys demonstrated a dramatic increase in satisfaction, moving from the seventy-ninth to the ninetieth percentile. There has also been a significant increase in letters, cards, and gifts given by patients to the staff on the patient-focused unit. And patients continue to state a preference for the unit.

Patient satisfaction may be due to increased continuity of care. Lakeland found that more than 60 percent of patients on the patient-focused units were seen exclusively by their primary physician throughout their hospitalization. The number of different personnel who interacted with patients during their stay at Lakeland dropped from twenty-seven to thirteen.

At Clarkson, patients commented on the advantages of decentralizing ancillary services. "I didn't have to go . . . down to the basement where the x-ray rooms are. It would take so long because you have to sit and wait. But, . . . on the ninth floor, in ten minutes, you are right back in your room again." Nursing staff and the care team are positive about the new system.

Reduced Length of Stay

Many hospitals applying the patient-focused approach have found that length of stay has decreased. At Robert Wood Johnson University Hospital, for example, lengths of stay have been sliced by 26 percent in the units where the system has been in operation the longest. At. St. Vincent, length of stay has been reduced by 17 percent on average for admissions projected at more than two days. At Lakeland, length of patient stay was sliced by 1.3 days on average for some treatments.

The reduced length of stay on the patient-focused orthopedics unit at Lee Memorial Medical Center resulted in a cost savings of $249,000 for the four-month period from June to September 1992. The following chart summarizes these savings:

	DRG 209	DRG 210	All other Diagnoses
Traditional Orthopedics	8.2 days	11.9 days	5.8 days
Redesigned Orthopedics	7.8 days	9.9 days	5.4 days

Improved Quality of Care

Patient-focused restructuring also contributes to improved quality of care and reduction of costly complications like pneumonia. Lee Memorial found a 50 percent reduction in medication errors, a 33 percent reduction in patient accidents, a 100 percent reduction in friction sores, a 50 percent reduction in intravenous problems, and an 83.3 percent reduction in ileus.

Productivity Improvements

Utilizing resources effectively is crucial for cost savings. By freeing up time previously devoted to unnecessary or redundant activities, the hospital can redeploy personnel so that direct patient-care time is increased. With the patient-focused approach, a hospital can simplify procedures, eliminate unnecessary documentation, and coordinate interdepartmental functions.

For example, some cost savings through productivity

improvements at Clarkson included: 47 percent reduction in medical documentation, 55 percent decline in scheduling and coordination time, 40 percent reduction in transportation time, 29 percent reduction in idle time, and the elimination of eleven employee classifications.

Turnaround Time. One of the most dramatic improvements resulting from decentralizing ancillary services is reduced turnaround time for tests. Lakeland, for example, found that turnaround time for routine tests fell from 157 minutes to 48 minutes: a 70 percent improvement. Diagnostic radiology procedures were simplified from forty steps taking 140 minutes to eight steps taking 28 minutes: an 80 percent reduction in turnaround time. Clarkson reported the elimination of twenty steps from the process for ordering laboratory tests. Another procedure that takes less time is turning over a bed between patients. At Vanderbilt University Medical Center, the four hours it took in the past was reduced to fifteen minutes.

Scheduling. Some patient-focused hospitals have also found that efficiency has improved through improved scheduling. For example, at Lee Memorial, the patient-focused plan led to increased awareness of problems in scheduling, followed by improvements in coordinating the schedules of interdependent departments.

Admissions Process. One dramatic improvement at Clarkson was the elimination of ten steps from the admissions process so that treatment could begin on an average of twenty-three minutes after the patient was admitted to the hospital; the previous time was eight hours. Also, the average time needed to begin implementing doctors' orders following admissions was cut by more than seven hours.

Charting-by-Exception. Patient-focused hospitals have reduced the volume of data in medical records by using charting-by-exception. This method involves the application of patient-care protocols. Charting-by-exception also results in a decrease in the amount of time that personnel spend in documentation activities. Vanderbilt realized a 31 percent decrease in documentation, while Clarkson reported a decrease of almost 50 percent.

Multiskilling. Cross-training staff to perform several tasks can result in dramatic cost savings. For example, at Lee Memorial Medical Center, training caregivers to perform phlebotomy for all laboratory draws allowed the hospital to eliminate a centralized phlebotomy area. As a result Lee Memorial was able to reduce staff by twenty-two full-time-equivalent employees (FTES), which at a cost of $7.01 per hour resulted in a savings of $320,777 per year. The net time added to caregivers' work was only ten minutes per shift.

Another example from Lee Memorial is training licensed caregivers to perform simple respiratory therapies for patients on the unit. The elimination of fifteen FTEs in the central respiratory-therapy department resulted in a savings of $410,000 per year (at $13.17 per hour). This change added only thirty minutes per shift. Training caregivers to perform EKGs eliminated four FTEs in the cardiology department for a savings of $65,395 at the rate of $7.86 per hour, and added one minute per caregiver shift.

Lee Memorial also reported that the implementation of a PYXIS system (a pharmaceutical ATM) for narcotics control significantly reduced the time for narcotics dispensing and inventory. The PYXIS system cost Lee Memorial approximately $25,000 per unit to implement. Use of this system was estimated to save eighteen minutes of caregiver time per shift.

Implementation of these various components of cross-training at Lee Memorial was projected to result in a net time savings of fifty-two minutes per caregiver per day. If fully realized, the savings resulting from reducing the current staffing by eighty-eight FTEs would be $2,355,724, calculated at $12.87 per hour.

Bedside Automation. Another aspect of patient-focused care that has resulted in both increased efficiency and increased savings is bedside automation. Bedside computer terminals create an electronic medical record of all aspects of a patient's hospitalization. Bedside automation eliminates both searching for the correct chart and writing information down on paper before transcribing it on a chart. Use of on-line information also has been found to increase accuracy (Chicago Health Executives Forum, 1991, p. 26).

Hospital Restructuring: A Radical Change

Hospital restructuring is a radical change in the fundamental process of delivering care. The goal is to improve productivity and quality by minimizing patient and caregiver movement within the hospital and by reducing the number of personnel interacting with each patient. However, the ultimate goal of this process is a much more fundamental one. The patient-focused hospital is a new paradigm, a new model of what the hospital can and ought to be.

At its core, patient-focused restructuring is about empowering patients and staff. It empowers patients because it places them at the center of hospital operations and offers continuity of care and fast, high-quality service. It empowers staff because nurses and technicians can feel in control of their jobs as the time they spend performing clerical tasks is substantially reduced. They can spend more of their time doing what they enjoy: caring for patients. Staff members also feel empowered because they know that they are providing humane and efficient services for their patients.

Although there are many advantages to restructuring services, it does require a substantial up-front investment in renovations. Also, cross-training necessitates costly initial and ongoing training and a possible short-term increase in turnover if staff cannot or will not adapt to the changes. Some argue that cross-training also compromises quality standards for ancillary staff.

Although the patient-focused model has definitely demonstrated some measurable benefits, further analysis must be done to evaluate the financial, personnel, and quality advantages of this model. As in any creative venture, risks are involved; however, this time of crisis in health care calls for bold ventures and the risk-taking that innovation demands.

In the next several chapters, we will continue our exploration of the patient-focused model by offering practical advice and suggestions for a step-by-step approach to implementation.

Chapter 3

Putting Healing
Back into Health Care

> The great error in the treatment of the human body is that
> physicians are ignorant of the whole. For the part can never be
> well unless the whole is well.
>
> Plato, cited by D. Jaffe, *Healing from Within**

Today, when we recognize a full 80 percent of diseases
as life-style related, it no longer makes sense to "fix" only the
physical problem. Kaiser (1992) uses the metaphor of the auto-
repair shop to describe the traditional hospital. Now, he says,
we need a new metaphor, where the focus is on the driver as
well as the car. It flies in the face of reason to continue fixing
only the automobile when the driver does not know how to drive.

When health care costs 54.6 percent of corporate pretax
profits and the average health plan costs $3,217 per employee
(1990, up 21.6 percent from 1989) (McManis and Pavia, 1991,
p. 17), employers, as well as private citizens, want more than
a repair job. In addition to long-term contracts that share the
risks and rewards of care and treatment, they want a focus on
health promotion, prevention, and patient empowerment.

With a patient-centered approach, patients and families
are encouraged and taught to be active participants in their care.
They learn about their illness, how their habits and patterns
may be contributing to their illness, and how to care for themselves. They are given alternatives, and their choices are incorporated into the treatment regime. With a hospital-centered ap-

---

*Dennis T. Jaffe, *Healing from Within: Psychological Techniques to Help the
Mind Heal the Body,* © 1980 by Alfred A. Knopf.

proach, care providers are trained in therapeutic presence, mind/body therapies, and the importance of family-centered care. Healing occurs because services come to the patient rather having the patient wheeled around the hospital wasting energy trying to fit into the schedules of some fifty or sixty different departments. Also, patient-centered care means continuity of care. As a result, patients and staff have an opportunity to get to know each other and to build relationships conducive to trust and learning. When we provide care from the patient's point of view, every person and every process within the environment play a part in enhancing the individual's unique healing potential.

This chapter presents a case for bringing healing back into health care. We begin by defining healing and its implications for patient care. Then, we explore how the interactions of patients and caregivers contribute to healing through patient and family empowerment and therapeutic presence. We then explore six mind/body therapies proven to facilitate healing, and, finally, we outline how the physical environment can enhance healing.

The essence of patient-centered care is reflected in the subtle difference between curing and healing. By and large the American health care system is focused on curing, on removing or eradicating the symptom or disease. Healing, however, makes one whole or well. It implies an integration of body, mind, and spirit. Whereas curing focuses on the disease or injury, healing focuses on the person experiencing the disease or injury. When the goal of treatment becomes healing, the context of care is changed. Success is no longer measured only by whether the diseased part is removed or a symptom is alleviated. When healing is the goal, the definition of success is expanded to include what the patient has learned and how well the patient is able to cope even though complete curing may not be possible. Healing implies that patient care operates on several levels: mental, emotional, and spiritual, as well as physical. It implies that patients are provided with the information and resources they need in order to use their experience of illness as an opportunity to learn about themselves and to move toward a sense of well-being.

Healing has many dimensions, all equally important. For example, the intervention of housekeepers as they intentionally clean the room and remove all clutter, dirt, and dust that may harbor bacteria and viruses contributes to a healing environment. Likewise, the intervention of cooks as they carefully cook the food at just the right temperatures and with the freshest ingredients promotes a patient's healing.

This shift in focus has profound implications for both patients and health care providers. For patients it means an active role as participants in their own care on all levels. For health care providers it means responsibility for providing the support systems and mechanisms that enhance the patient's unique healing potential. The patient becomes the focus of care rather than the system, the disease, or the injury. When the patient is the center of care, empowering patients and families becomes a primary responsibility of all the health care team members.

Patient and Family Empowerment

Jevin (1991) defines empowerment as the sense that one is able to influence one's own life. Studies support the clinical observation that being able to influence one's life is important for the management of and recovery from disease. Ultimately, patients are responsible for their own lives. Yet the power of the hospital system to inhibit or enhance healing and recovery is considerable. Unfortunately, the traditional hospital experience often disempowers patients and families by reducing the amount of control they have while hospitalized. For example, removing personal items and serving meals or giving medications according to someone else's schedule result in patients' loss of identity. By substituting formulas for personalized care, we treat patients as cases rather than individuals. Even though their physical limitations may require some patients to accept a degree of dependence, their role does not have to be a completely passive one. On the contrary, research indicates that the most effective way to promote healing is for patients to become active participants in their care (Speedling and Rosenberg, 1986).

First, patients who are invited to be active participants in their care are far more likely to disclose pertinent information than those who are not involved. Even with all the technology of modern medicine, the most skilled clinician must rely on the quality of the patient's information to know what is wrong and how to help. This information has a direct influence on the ability of physicians and staff to provide quality care. Planetree in San Francisco, for example, includes a team meeting with patient, family, physician, and nurse as part of the admissions process (Jenna, 1986a). During this meeting, patients and their family are invited to identify their goals and participate in developing their plan of care. Planetree also involves patients throughout their hospital stay by encouraging them to write their own progress notes in their medical record.

Second, hospitalization can be viewed as a socialization experience that helps patients adapt to life with a chronic illness (Speedling and Rosenberg, 1986). In order for this adaptation to occur, patients must understand and accept the reasons for the treatment plan as well as develop new knowledge and skills to cope with their condition. Patients and their family must be active participants in this process in order to demonstrate their understanding and to learn skills that can often be quite complex. The New York University Medical Center's Cooperative Care Unit (Grieco and others, 1990) encourages this participation by having live-in family members or friends act as "care partners" for patients. Their model emphasizes education in order to encourage full involvement by patient and family in care during hospitalization, so that both will be prepared to manage care at home after discharge. The Cooperative Care Unit reports shorter lengths of stay and a 37.5 percent cost savings per hospitalization as compared with the traditional hospital. In addition, patient and family learning and satisfaction are enhanced.

Third, the experience of illness and hospitalization is a crisis for both patients and their families. Patients often ask themselves or others such questions as "How did I get to this point in my life?" and "Why is this happening to me?" Even though highly stressful, this time of crisis is also rich in opportunity for patients to identify unmet needs and make needed life-style changes. As one patient put it, "My back was against the wall. I couldn't deny it any longer. When the doctor gave me the report and told me what my options were, I knew it was up to me. I had to stop drinking and I had to come clean with my relationship with Sue. It was time to start living my life." When care providers encourage patients to explore these questions, the choices they make, and the options available to them, patients are empowered to make new choices that enrich and enhance their health and well-being.

Fourth, patients who are empowered with choices and information generally have better outcomes than those who are not. For example, a serious aftermath of coronary bypass surgery that affects approximately 30 percent of patients is depression. Depression is a serious disorder; it retards recovery, lowers treatment compliance, and increases the length of stay in the hospital. Pimm (1991) found that providing crisis intervention to patients during their hospital stay and for eight weeks after discharge significantly lowered depression scores compared with those of a nonintervention group. These differences between group scores increased over time for as long as three years after surgery. Even more important, studies show that the use of bibliotherapy (giving patients a carefully designed book describing the surgical experience and feelings they might have) proved equally as effective as crisis intervention by a therapist. Use of the book alone lowered depression scores. Research by Egbert and others (1964) demonstrated that providing patients with information about what to expect after their surgery and how they could participate in their recovery resulted in reduced length of hospital stays and decreased the need for narcotics.

Also, research consistently shows that persons who have no information regarding the timing, frequency, and onset of painful experiences have more pain, greater physiological reactions, and more impairment in the performance of tasks than people who are informed (as cited by Taylor, 1979). One poignant example of the importance of informing patients about discomfort associated with procedures is this excerpt from a letter by a young child to her physician. "I want you to know you should never lie to people. You told me it wouldn't hurt when you took off my bandage. It hurt alot, and I will never trust you again. I know I will never see you again, but maybe you will remember this the next time you take off someone's bandage."

The lack of empowerment can actually compromise patients' health. Too often, hospitalized patients lose the ability to perform functions they were able to perform before entering the hospital. Many patients fear hospitalization for this reason. Perhaps this loss occurs most often with chronically ill and elderly patients. Many times, well-intended caregivers do too much for patients or fail to inform them and involve them in decision making. Caregivers often feel that they do not have enough time and that it is quicker to do things for patients instead of waiting for patients to do them in their own time and on their own schedule.

Being unable to do things for themselves, lack of information, and the inability to control events may lead to patients' developing a sense of helplessness. Helplessness is a state of passivity and an inability to take charge of one's condition. Seligman (1975) reports numerous studies showing that individuals lose their ability to learn in environments where they lose their ability to control events. His research demonstrates that helplessness can lead to depression. Furthermore, patients can become conditioned to helplessness, leading to what Seligman calls "learned helplessness." Learned helplessness can persist even after conditions change to allow personal control—for example, after a patient returns home after hospitalization. A common occurrence in many hospitals is that elderly people require nursing-home placement after hospitalization, even though they were active and independent before.

However, the main culprit in encouraging helplessness and dependence is the hospital system itself. The traditional hospital system is based on the completion of tasks. Care is provided over eight-hour shifts, and caregivers are focused on completing their assigned tasks in the allotted time. Traditionally, little thought is given to the fact that from a patient's point of view, hospitalization is but one point in a whole continuum of health. Without a patient-centered philosophy, the emphasis on efficiency means that staff members are rewarded for completing tasks during their shifts instead of for encouraging patient independence and teaching patients how to maintain their own health and care for themselves.

Kobasa (1979), a well-known researcher, has summarized the vital role of empowerment in her groundbreaking studies. She identifies three recurring personality characteristics of people who cope well with stress. The first, control, is the absence of powerlessness. It is a belief that one can influence one's own experience. The second is commitment, the ability to feel involved and to have a sense of meaning for one's life. The third is a sense of challenge, a perception of approaching change or problems as an opportunity for learning and personal growth. Kobasa calls these three characteristics hardiness factors.

Pollock (1989) added to Kobasa's research by applying these hardiness characteristics to patients' ability to adapt to health problems. She recommends the use of this health-related hardiness research for guiding nursing interventions in patient care. Such a program includes helping and encouraging patients to be active participants in their care by empowering them with information, offering them choices, and integrating their goals, choices, and decisions into their plan of care. It also includes helping patients and their family to use their illness or injury as an opportunity for increasing understanding of themselves and identifying needed life-style changes.

For example, many patients who have cancer talk of how the experience changed and enhanced their life. LeShan (1989) reports in his book, *Cancer as a Turning Point,* how he helps patients use their disease as an opportunity for increased understanding of their needs and fulfillment of their dreams. He explains his approach: "What is right with this person? . . . What is . . . his unique song to sing so that when he is singing it he is glad to get up in the morning? . . . How can we work together to find these ways of being, relating, and creating? What has blocked their perception and/or expression in the past? How can we work together so that the person moves more and more in this direction?" (p. 537). LeShan reports that some cancer patients have undergone tumor regression and increased the length of their lives as a result of his approach (as cited in U.S. Congress, 1990).

Therapeutic Presence

Because hospitals are a service industry, their product exists in the people they employ. When viewed in this way, the conscious presence of care providers is an important concern. Therapeutic presence can be defined as the conscious intention to be present for another in a helpful or healing way. It is based on a commitment to help others and involves a lifelong commitment to self-development. In this section, we will explore therapeutic presence and outline three key elements of this concept: continuity of care, the placebo effect, and the consciousness of the care provider.

Before we examine these elements, try this exercise: Close your eyes and recall an experience you or a loved one has had as a hospitalized patient. Jot down your key memories and what you perceived as quality care. Now review what you have written.

If you are like most people you relate the quality of your care to the quality of your relationship with your care providers. The evidence for the importance of the personal characteristics of caregivers and their interpersonal skills in patient satisfaction and outcome is considerable (Roter, Hall, and Katz, 1988; Suchman and Matthews, 1988; Kaplan, Greenfield, and Ware, 1989; Rowland-Morin and Carroll, 1990; and Bertakis, Roter, and Putman, 1991). Consistently, patients value warmth, compassion, and attention to the needs of their whole person. For example, Di Matteo and Hays (1980) report that patient satisfaction with physicians is more likely to be influenced by the way their psychosocial needs are met than by their perceptions of their physician's competence.

Continuity of Care

The most vital component in any relationship is being there for the other person, both physically and mentally. As self-evident as this requirement may seem, it is often missing in patient care in traditional hospitals. One of the most common complaints of patients and families is "I never see the same face twice." It is difficult to form a therapeutic, trusting relationship when, as the average hospital reports, a patient typically sees fifty-five different caregivers during a three-day stay (Lathrop, 1991). Patients and staff are constantly having to get to know each other and starting from scratch in identifying needs and preferences. Everyone seems to agree that continuity is an important component of quality care. However, many factors interfere with this important goal. Key among these factors are abrupt changes in patient census, most often as a result of short lengths of stay and a physician-driven surgery schedule; specialization and the presence of numerous departments; and the lack of a patient-centered care philosophy. Patient-centered restructuring can help dramatically by creating focus units.

On a focus unit patients with similar and predicable needs are grouped together. Needed ancillary services are placed on the unit, and staff members are cross-trained so that patients interact with the same caregivers. Because of the similarity of patient needs, staffing and census are more predictable than on a traditional hospital floor. As a result, team members can be consistently assigned to their patients rather than to their various departments. For example, an orthopedic unit might include a physical therapist as a permanent member of the team. Attention also is paid to how the surgery schedule affects patient care both postoperatively and preoperatively. Surgeries can then be scheduled with thought for patients' long-range needs such as the availability of staff. We will say more about these strategies in Chapters Four and Five.

The Placebo Effect

Unfortunately, in the past the placebo (Latin for "I shall please") was used primarily to determine whether patients were telling the truth about their pain. The physician would order an injection of normal saline (the placebo), and if the patient reported pain relief, he was privately scoffed at and labeled a malingerer. Now we know that the placebo effect is based on the person's positive expectant belief that the medication or treatment will work.

Throughout history, the major cause of healing may have been the patient's own positive expectations and beliefs. It is now generally agreed that nearly every interaction between care provider (physician, nurse, therapist, or any other helper) and a patient has some component of the placebo built into it (O'Regan, 1985). Positive suggestion can enhance the effects of treatments and create beneficial results from otherwise useless treatments. Consistently, research studies show that placebos are effective in about one-third of all cases (Jaffee, 1980). If the patient believes the treatment or medication will help, it is likely to help.

For example, Beecher (1955) analyzed data from fifteen studies involving 1,082 patients with conditions as varied as headache, anxiety, severe postoperative pain, and the common cold. He found placebos had a significant effect in treating 35 percent of these conditions. Beecher also reviewed two double-blind studies indicating that surgery can act as a placebo. Surgeons who were optimistic that internal ligation (tying off) of the mammary artery would relieve angina (heart pain) reported significant pain relief of up to 75 percent. Surgeons more skeptical of the possibility of success reported their patients had much less pain relief. Dr. Leonard Cobb and colleagues (as cited by Hurley, 1985) tested this approach by studying the effects of performing a fake surgery. In this study skin incisions alone were made. No arteries were tied off. They found that 43 percent of the patients receiving the fake operation reported improvement, whereas only 32 percent of patients having the ligation reported improvement. They also found that the placebo surgery reduced patients' need for nitroglycerine for pain and increased their ability to exercise and to work.

Another interesting review of the power of the placebo effect is reported by Evans (1984). After reviewing placebo research from 1959 to 1974, he found that 36 percent of patients experience over 30 percent relief of pain through the use of placebos. He also found that the potency of the drug mattered little. For example, placebos were 54 percent as effective as aspirin in nine double-blind studies and 56 percent as effective as morphine (a potent narcotic) in six double-blind studies.

However, the placebo effect has the power to hinder patient comfort and recovery if used in a negative way. Larkin (1985) reports how, as a nurse, she spends much of her time countering nontherapeutic suggestions. Well-intentioned health care providers, unaware of the importance of how they present treatments and activities to patients, may actually worsen their pain or increase complications.

What does this mean in practical terms? Here are some examples from my (Nancy Moore) experience of how staff can counter nontherapeutic suggestions. In one case, I arrived just in time to help Tommy turn. Tommy's bicycle accident left him with a fractured back and two broken legs. Tommy's nurse began the procedure by saying, "This is really going to hurt." Tommy winced, stiffened, and began to cry. I countered this nontherapeutic suggestion by saying, "It's always amazing to me how easily and comfortably patients can turn when they do the following things. Watch me, Tommy, and do what I do. Take three deep breaths. Put your arm over your chest. I will support your back and leg as Cindy gently turns you." Tommy stopped crying, and the procedure was completed with a minimum of discomfort.

In another case Sally had a severe burn on her right arm. The doctor rushed into Sally's room. "Get the gelfoam. I'm going to change the dressing and it will bleed like hell." Sally's eyes grew big and she began to cry. While her nurse went for the supplies needed for the dressing change, I talked to Sally. "You know, Sally, the body just knows so well how to heal. It knows how to bleed in just the right amount to cleanse your burn and allow the skin to grow. You can help your body by taking a few good breaths, breathing oxygen into these cells. That's good now." As the doctor changed the dressing, we played her favorite song, and Sally squeezed my hand every time it hurt while she breathed in the healing oxygen. The procedure was completed without the need for gelfoam to stop the bleeding.

Consciousness of the Care Provider

As mentioned earlier, therapeutic presence is the conscious intention to be present for another in a healing or helpful way.

This process highlights the importance of encouraging and helping care providers to enhance their own health and potential. Truly, you cannot give what you do not have.

Lynch (1979) provides an interesting review of studies supporting the effects of human interaction on health. One study demonstrated that holding a patient's hand to take a pulse may suppress heart irregularities. Other studies have linked changes in blood chemistry to human companionship. For example, Glaser and others (1987) compared thirty-four family caregivers of Alzheimer's disease patients to thirty-four control subjects. They found that the constant stress endured by these caregivers resulted in lower percentages of important factors in the immune system, such as helper T cells, total T cells, helper/suppressor T-cell ratios, and natural killer (NK) cells. Even more interesting was their finding that caregivers who were involved in support groups showed significantly higher percentages of NK cells, important for immune-system functioning, than those not involved in support groups. Furthermore, in his work with cancer patients, LeShan (1989) relates that therapy "depends on a real 'encounter,' a real contact between therapist and client. The therapist must, moreover, care intensely, believe in the importance of and be involved in the special growth, the individual becoming, of the hospital" (p. 38).

Although the assumption has been that patients undergoing surgery are asleep so it really does not matter what care providers say, there is evidence to the contrary. Cheek (1959) and Levinson (1965) document that under hypnosis patients can recall statements made during surgery by the operating team. Cheek has successfully used hypnosis and ventilation therapy to treat unexplained postoperative anxiety and depression, which he attributes to remarks made during surgery. This groundbreaking work for humanizing the process of surgery continues with researchers and therapists such as Bennett (1985), E. Anderson (1987), and Barber (1984).

At the Second National Conference on the Psychology of Health, Immunity and Disease, Bennett (1990) reminded participants that patients under anesthesia are not asleep, they are unconscious. When people are unconscious their auditory system is still active and even though they do not consciously remember what is heard, they can still learn. As Bennett warns, "The real issue is: what is learned during surgery persists later but is not identified by the patient as resulting from the intraoperative period" (p. 2). Therefore, care providers bear responsibility for using this time as an opportunity to provide therapeutic messages and healing comments for patient recovery.

I have noted the effects of my state of consciousness on patients' recovery. For example, I recall entering a patient's room while tense and thinking of an upsetting situation I had just encountered. The patient immediately sensed that I was not present for her. She became agitated and abruptly asked me to leave her room. However, I also recall taking a few deep breaths before entering another patient's room and consciously thinking of being present for her. I entered in a relaxed state and focused on the patient and her needs. As I sat in a chair, I listened intently to her description of her frustration with her failure to recover from her surgery. She began to cry, and I softly held her hand. She thanked me for being there for her. Later, as I passed her in the hall, she said, "You don't know how much your taking the time to be with me yesterday helped. It seemed to get me over the hump. My doctor says I can go home tomorrow."

Care providers are expert facilitators who are responsible for creating an experience that optimizes the patient's unique healing potential. Kaiser (1991d) describes patient-centered care as a dramaturgic event, an improvisational theater, with physicians, nurses, and others as actors in the sense that they are responsible for creating an experience that encourages, empowers, and utilizes the patient's own belief system to facilitate healing.

The following stories describe a negative, then a positive, way of relating to patients. Imagine you are a patient recovering from surgery. You call for pain medication. A nurse rushes into your room and abruptly exclaims, "What do you want?" You reply, and she leaves. When she returns, she abruptly gives you the medication and scurries out of the room.

Now, imagine that you call for pain medication. This time as the nurse enters she caringly inquires about your pain. She shows you how to take a few deep breaths for some immediate relief. She replies, "I will return in a few moments with a very effective medication for your pain." When she returns she tells you the name of the medication and how it works as she administers it. She says, "This medication will make you more comfortable." She also inquires whether she can do anything else to increase your comfort. She leaves the room while informing you she will check back in about thirty minutes and asking you to call if you require anything in the interim. Both nurses administered the medication. Yet the patient's experience, both physiologically and psychologically, will be quite different.

Mind/Body Therapies

Specialists from a variety of fields (stress, psychoneuroimmunology, neuroendocrinology, molecular biology, and others) have demonstrated that thoughts, images, and feelings have biochemical counterparts that have direct effects on the physical body. This mind/body connection has been established since the pioneering work of Hans Selye. Selye demonstrated that stress, a mental phenomenon, leads to physical changes in the body, such as increased heart rate, sweating, increased stress hormones in the blood, and decreased functioning of the immune system. Other, psychological effects of stress include anxiety, depression, and a sense of helplessness. The connection of mind and body is now so clear that it no longer seems appropriate to segregate the body and mind into separate fields of study. For this reason, we are witnessing the advent of a new discipline of medicine: psychoneuroimmunology.

Mind/body therapies treat the patient as a whole person. They add to patient empowerment because once patients learn them they can use them on their own. Also, because they utilize the person's innate resources, there are no undesirable side effects. In this section we will explore six such therapies: relaxation training, guided imagery and visualization, meditation, therapeutic touch, massage, and counseling.

Relaxation Training

The relaxed state can be thought of as a healing state. When the body is relaxed, it is in its most balanced state: heart rate is normal, breathing is full and regular, the mind is peaceful, and the body systems, including the immune system, function at their best. Benson (1975) describes this psychophysiological state as the relaxation response. During the relaxation response, pulse, blood pressure, respiration, oxygen consumption, carbon dioxide production, muscle tone, and metabolic rate are all decreased. When patients are relaxed, they have a heightened ability to concentrate, are receptive to positive suggestion, and feel peaceful. The following are a few quick and easy relaxation methods that hospital staff can learn on their own, then teach to others (DiMotto, 1984).

Full-Body Relaxation. This method involves focusing on different parts of the body, noticing any tension, then replacing it with relaxation. DiMotto recommends that this exercise be done as part of the bath as long as the patient is willing. For example, the nurse can instruct the patient to notice any tension as she washes the arm. Then she instructs the patient to "breathe in warmth and relaxation to this arm and exhale tension." During drying, the patient is instructed to "notice the warmth and relaxation you now feel in this arm" (p. 755). These instructions are repeated throughout the bath. After practicing a few times, patients can generally do this exercise themselves.

Modified Autogenic Relaxation. Relaxation from this method is achieved through a series of self-statements (autosuggestions) about different body functions. Patients assume a relaxed position, slowly inhaling and exhaling as they repeat a series of phrases identifying different areas of the body. Patients inhale as they identify a body part and exhale while describing a relaxed feeling. As with all relaxation exercises, repetition leads to thorough and quick results. DiMotto recommends this method in the treatment of asthma, hyperventilation, cold hands and feet, high blood pressure, headache, and ulcers.

Ten-Second Relaxation. A number of quick, effective exercises can be used by patients experiencing incisional pain and anxiety. DiMotto describes one of them: "Eyes open, let your lower jaw drop as if you are starting to yawn. Rest your tongue on the bottom of your mouth. . . . Breathe slowly and rhythmically through your mouth: inhale, exhale, then rest. Do not form or even think of words" (p. 757).

Benson and Stuart (1992) teach clients at the Mind/Body Medical Clinic of New England Deaconess Hospital and Harvard Medical School similar exercises called "minis." These exercises range from taking a few conscious breaths to sitting quietly for several minutes. Research shows that patients using these exercises use fewer narcotics after surgery and report less pain than those not using them.

Music. Patients often identify listening to music as a preferred method of relaxation. Patients can be encouraged to choose their own music. However, the Largo movements of classical music are often most effective in promoting relaxation because their rhythmic cycle of sixty beats per minute tend to synchronize with the human biological rhythm resulting in deeper relaxation. Don G. Campbell (as cited by Kaiser, 1991f), founder and director of the Institute for Music, Health and Education in Boulder, Colorado, is a pioneer in the application of therapeutic sound. He teaches that music affects the body's rhythms by altering the pulse rate, blood pressure, brain waves, and respiration patterns. Also, he finds that having patients listen to slow classical music through headphones thirty minutes before an operation reduces the amount of anesthesia needed by about 30 percent. He says, "The sound environment of the hospital can be foreign at best and jarring or unconducive to healing at worst" (p. 6). As part of a planned healing environment, he recommends quality sound systems with individual headsets for patients.

In addition, relaxation can be combined with guided imagery and visualization to further enhance the patient's own natural healing potential.

Guided Imagery and Visualization

The Simontons (Simonton, Simonton, and Creighton, 1978), pioneers in the use of imagery in the treatment of cancer, use guided imagery and visualization to strengthen the immune system and perhaps even to alter the course of a disease. Hall (1982) supports the Simontons' work with his findings that patients using positive-imagery techniques experience an increase in disease-fighting lymphocytes and hormone levels known to augment the immune system. Although their work initially generated a great deal of controversy, their methods are now widely used in most traditional medical establishments along with conventional treatments.

Jaffee (1980) reports how an orthopedic surgeon, Robert Swearingen, uses these methods. While working in an emergency room located near a ski resort, Swearingen noticed that certain ski-patrol members brought in patients who were consistently much easier to care for and required less pain medication. After investigating, he found that these ski-patrol members instinctively helped their patients relax. After Swearingen taught all the ski-patrol members relaxation skills, he found a 50 percent decrease in the use of pain medication. When setting fractures, he also began using imagery exercises to help patients control the pain. In addition, he explained how the bone heals and suggested that patients visualize this process during their recovery. Swearingen found that the patients using imagery were ready for cast removal in about 30 percent less time than those who did not use it.

Although there is no conclusive evidence about how visualization works, we do know it improves the healing process by reducing pain and giving patients some control.

Meditation

Current research shows that using meditation as a therapeutic tool helps reduce blood pressure (Benson, 1975); reduces the incidence of disease (Orme-Johnson and Schneider, 1987); lowers cholesterol levels (Cooper and Aygen, 1970); reduces stress and anxiety (Bruning and Frew, 1987); improves the ability to breathe and decreases the symptoms of asthma (Honsberger and Wilson, 1973); enhances the beneficial effects of treatment for heart disease and cancer (Ornish, 1990); and improves health factors related to the aging process (Orme-Johnson and Schneider, 1987). Through the practice of meditation, patients can learn to detach themselves from passing thoughts that distract the mind or lead to identification with pain or suffering. Meditation helps patients increase awareness and experience states of tranquility and peace.

Meditation is a process of focusing the mind on a simple activity or process. It can be learned in a few moments, although it requires continued and regular practice, ideally ten to twenty minutes once or twice a day, to be truly mastered.

The staff of the Mind/Body Medical Institute of New England Deaconess Hospital and Harvard Medical School use meditation to elicit the relaxation response by teaching clients to turn their attention inward, concentrating on a repetitive focus such as breathing or on a word or on a prayer. According to Benson and Stuart (1992), they say to clients, "As you practice the relaxation response with meditation, you will have moments of entering quieter states quite removed from the stressful levels of activity that make up most of your daily life. In these moments of profound rest, you may experience greater awareness, enhanced self-esteem, and a deepening of your commitment to your health" (p. 48).

Nearly all forms of meditation are modifications of these basic steps:

1. Find a quiet place and sit comfortably with your spine as straight as possible.
2. Begin by focusing inward on your breathing or on a sensation or on a word or phrase.
3. Become aware of your body, scan your whole physical being, noticing how it feels.
4. Gradually begin relaxing your body, going deeper and deeper into a state of relaxation allowing yourself to experience a sense of peace.
5. If distracting thoughts come in your mind simply observe them like bubbles in a river or a passing stream. When your mind wanders, gently return your focus to your breathing or feeling of peace and relaxation or to a simple phrase or prayer.
6. After ten to twenty minutes, gradually return to your normal state of awareness.

Counseling

Counseling can be defined as an interactive process between the patient and care provider that influences the patient's feelings, attitudes, thoughts, and action. Nurses and other caregivers contribute to patient healing when they help patients express thoughts and feelings as well as adjust to and learn from their illness.

The American Hospital Association (1990) estimates that 25 percent of those hospitalized have alcohol-related problems. This percentage does not include patients with illnesses complicated by other substance abuse. This shocking statistic, combined with the established fact that eleven of the fourteen leading causes of death are subject to the influence of life-style factors (R. Anderson, 1987), indicates the need for hospitals to incorporate counseling methods into their therapeutic regimes. Despite substantial research supporting the efficacy of counseling approaches, the American health care system is slow to integrate them into the day-to-day care of patients.

The Integrated Medical Unit of Washoe Medical Center in Reno integrates a counseling approach into all interactions with patients. Utilizing a "healing questionnaire," as a guide, staff members help patients and families address the depression, anxiety, fear, grief and loss, life-style adjustments, family issues, issues of addiction, and spiritual distress that often accompany illness. The nurses have special training in utilizing every conversation as an intervention in healing. Washoe also includes the family and integrates group processes such as a self-help recovery model into the therapeutic regime.

Other hospitals, recognizing the futility of treating only the physical manifestation of disease or injury, are beginning to address underlying psychological issues. For example, in Portland, Oregon, Emanuel Hospital instituted a chemical-dependency assessment for all trauma patients with a blood alcohol level above the legal limit. They found that 31 percent were alcoholic and 41 percent were both alcoholic and drug dependent. "Roughly 72 percent of trauma patients with raised alcohol levels are substance abusers," says Dr. Anthony Borzotta. "For years we have known that abusers cause accidents, but the physician community ignored it, . . . ignored a medical condition that often resulted in injury" (as cited in "Doing the Right Thing," 1991, p. 3). As part of their program, a chemical-dependency evaluator sees patients as soon as they are stable. The evaluator says, "Though I can't influence everyone to seek treatment, I firmly believe that I plant a seed. . . . They will never use alcohol or drugs again without knowing that it is destructive. . . . They begin to realize that their accident was a wake up call, and that making their future better is in their hands" (p. 3).

As a part of a counseling approach, it is also important to encourage patients to tell their illness or trauma story. Pennebaker (1990) found that both verbal expression and simply writing about thoughts and feelings related to traumatic experiences heightened immune function. Bressler (1984) of the UCLA Pain Center reports that such storytelling is one of his most powerful interventions. "Sometimes, once the patient has expressed his story fully, the pain subsides. As a result, the treatment has been completed."

Recently, I was called to work with a patient suffering from lung cancer. As we talked, he had to rest frequently because of the difficulty he had in breathing. He talked of a sense of fear and deep sadness. As he focused on his feelings and recalled the loss of his father ten years ago, he began sobbing, expressing his deep grief over his loss. This was the first time he had acknowledged his grief. In the past he had never given himself permission to cry. He had been taught as a child that boys do not cry, a message reinforced by our society. He reported that this release of long pent-up emotion was beneficial. He felt lighter and felt he had more space to breathe. He chose to continue in counseling on an outpatient basis.

Group therapy is another approach that has proven helpful in patient recovery. David Spiegel and colleagues (as cited in U.S. Congress, 1990) found that psychotherapy, consisting of weekly ninety-minute supportive group sessions, and teaching self-hypnosis for pain control improved survival and quality of life for patients with metastatic breast cancer. Women with breast cancer who underwent group psychotherapy lived an average of 36.6 months after surgery as compared with women in a control group, who lived only 18.9 months after surgery. Also, Spiegel found that psychotherapy reduced anxiety, depression, and pain. The investigators believe support groups help patients mobilize their resources, improving compliance with conventional treatment.

Therapeutic Touch

Touch has been used in healing since ancient times. Therapeutic Touch (Krieger, Peper, and Ancoli, 1979) is a way of acting as an instrument of healing in the sense of integrating body, mind, and spirit. The focus is on the process of balancing the energies of the total person rather than on the treatment of a disease (Macrae, 1990).

There have been seventeen doctoral dissertations and nine postdoctoral studies completed on the subject of Therapeutic Touch as well as innumerable master's theses and clinical studies. One of these studies was done by Heidt (1979), who investigated the use of Therapeutic Touch to treat anxiety in ninety cardiovascular patients. She found a significant decrease in anxiety in the group receiving Therapeutic Touch as compared with control groups receiving casual touch and no touch. Many other studies also support the use of Therapeutic Touch in relieving anxiety and pain (Heidt, 1981; Randolph, 1984; Quinn, 1982; and Meehan, 1985).

Therapeutic Touch is based on the belief that human beings are fundamentally energy, and when people are ill, upset, or injured, their energy pattern becomes imbalanced or depleted. This concept is supported by the relativistic quantum-field theories of modern physics. Findings in quantum physics indicate that energy fields are the basic organizing forces of the universe. In explaining the energy field that practitioners feel during the practice of Therapeutic Touch, we can draw on the fact that the human body functions through the use of electricity. There is a constant flow of positively and negatively charged ions through our cell membranes. This electrical flow is detected when we measure the activity of the heart through EKGs or of brain waves through electroencephalograms or of muscle activity with electromyograms. Another way the human energy field is demonstrated is through the use of kirlian photography, which reveals a soft light surrounding life forms.

Through using Therapeutic Touch, practitioners are able to feel and direct the human energy field with their hands. Using their hands, they assess the body for areas of energy imbalance or depletion. Once these areas are identified, treatment can begin. The treatment consists of rebalancing the flow of energy and directing healing energy to areas that are depleted by moving the hands a few inches above the body. When the field becomes balanced and even, the treatment is completed, and the patient is asked to rest for fifteen to twenty minutes. Key to the practice of Therapeutic Touch is the process of becoming centered and focused on the patient with the positive intention to help or heal. Many nurses report this process has helped them become more calm and focused in all their care than they were previously.

As a Therapeutic-Touch practitioner for more than eight years, I have found it to be a helpful method in relieving patients' pain and anxiety. For some, the relief is quite dramatic, even after conventional methods have failed; for others, the effects are not as noticeable. Yet almost everyone reports some relaxation or pain relief (or both) as a result of the intervention.

At this time, Therapeutic Touch is quite controversial because it derives from the ancient healing practice of "laying on of hands" and because physicians fear it will be used as a replacement for medical therapies. The developers of Therapeutic Touch, Delores Krieger and Dora Kunz, teach that although Therapeutic Touch is a natural process that anyone can learn, it is not a replacement for medical approaches. It is one more tool for promoting a person's healing. Krieger (1988) has taught over 17,000 health professionals how to use Therapeutic Touch in this way. With a patient-centered philosophy, whether medical practitioners accept that Therapeutic Touch works is not the issue. It helps patients. The essence of patient-centered care is to move beyond established paradigms and to look at those factors that contribute to meeting patients' needs and healing.

Massage

"It is a whole other world to have a massage. . . . We so often cut ourselves off from the foundation of healing. Massage is not an ending, but a beginning—an education to tuning inside and listening to yourself. . . . Massage facilitates a slowing down of the mind. . . . Massage is a balance to so many other things that happen in the hospital" (as cited by Kaiser, 1991a, p. 3). These are the words of Karen Gibson, a nurse and massage therapist at Boulder Community Hospital in Colorado. Gibson's massage-therapy department is one of the leading hospital-based programs in the country. It provides massage on a consultation basis when requested by patients, physicians, or nurses and serves as a training site for students of the Boulder School of Massage.

Primary areas for the use of massage are oncology and obstetrics. Gibson finds that cancer patients are particularly in need of this type of therapy. "Many people in the hospital are just lying there, and they don't think they are doing anything to help themselves get well. . . . I teach them how to bring energy into their hands. . . . I might ask [a patient] to imagine warmth and love flowing from her heart down her arm and into her hands—with her hands placed on the surface area of where the tumor lies. Some people come to hate their illness and their bodies. I ask them, 'How can you help heal what you hate?'" (quoted in Kaiser, 1991e, p. 4). The use of massage in obstetrics has the potential for being an attractive marketing tool. Although the trend toward jacuzzis and fancy decors in obstetrics departments is nice, Gibson points out that a massage may be more attractive after delivering a baby.

Another way to improve obstetrical care is through neonatal massage. Patti Douglas, a certified massage therapist at Saint Luke's Medical Center in Denver, teaches infant massage to nurses and parents of premature babies. "I observe a high level of satisfaction in nurses when they provide massage and see the response from infants" (quoted in Kaiser, 1991a, p. 5). In addition, she teaches parents how to intentionally touch their premature infants. These parents often feel helpless and afraid in the high-tech atmosphere of the neonatal intensive-care nursery. She finds infant massage helps them continue the bonding process.

Other hospitals that are using massage include Planetree at California Pacific Medical Center in San Francisco and HCA Wesley Medical Center in Wichita, Kansas. These programs offer massage to help facilitate healing in patients who are touch-deprived or in need of comfort for relief of pain, tension, sleeplessness, or anxiety. Although massage is not reimbursed by third-party payers, these hospitals have been able to continue offering the service as a result of the use of volunteers and alliances with massage-therapy schools.

With a patient-centered approach, patients' preferences for and patterns of relaxation are explored, and special attention is paid to the provision of rest. Staff members are trained in a variety of therapies such as relaxation techniques, counseling skills, guided imagery, visualization, and therapeutic touch. Patients are given alternatives, and their choices are incorporated into their treatment plan.

Physical Environment

"Most hospitals are dismally inhospitable. A weakened patient and traumatized family are greeted by harsh lights and cold stainless steel, labyrinths of white corridors, thumping equipment, and acrid, mysterious smells. The sick rarely have access to information, privacy or a place for quiet talk and grieving. The resulting sense of anxiety and helplessness is the worst imaginable to promote healing" (Horn, 1991, p. 48). Patient-centered design and architecture do more than meet codes and cost and efficiency standards. They promote patient well-being; they complement the efforts of physicians and nurses and foster the process of healing and recovery. These results are possible because designs are created from the patient's point of view. These designs minimize the inherent stress of hospitalization, promote patient self-control of the environment, create a home-like atmosphere, and promote healing through the use of the person's sensory systems. (We will take a closer look at the role of the environment in healing in Chapter Six.)

Minimizing Stress

Remember the last time you were a patient in the hospital. Recall how you felt on arrival, as you entered your room, and during your hospital stay. If you are like most people, you probably felt a slight sense of anxiety, with a quickening of your breath and heartbeat. No matter how you look at it, illness and hospitalization are stressful experiences. Stress has both psychological and physiological components that work against healing. As a result, stress can impair healing and contribute to patients' failure to follow medical instructions. Carpman, Grant, and Simmons (1986) describe ways that design and architecture can be used to reduce stress. They identify these patient-centered approaches as promoting "wayfinding," physical comfort, regulation of social contact, and symbolic meaning.

Wayfinding. Typical in many hospitals is the lost visitor or patient searching for the laboratory, admitting office, or some other destination. Carpman, Grant, and Simmons (1986) found that the terminology used on signs is extremely important. Their research indicates that some terms that are obvious to medical personnel, such as "internal medicine" and "nuclear medicine," may cause confusion and fear in consumers. They recommend the use of clear, plain, patient-centered language. Other helpful suggestions include the use of "you-are-here" maps, an easily accessible information desk, distinctive interior landmarks (artwork or architectural features), and the use of printed materials.

Physical Comfort. One of the most frequent criticisms of hospitals is they devalue rest and comfort in the healing and recovery process. Cousins (1979) eloquently challenged the traditional system when he signed himself out of the hospital during a grave illness. Later, he recovered in a hotel room using a library of funny videos and tapes. In my experience, patients frequently complain about discomfort from mattresses, chairs, and breezy hospital attire. Patient-centered healing calls for attention to comfort in every aspect of design, including color choices, lighting, furnishings, room design, hospital attire, and placement of controls.

Regulation of Social Contact. Although the need for privacy is obvious, most observers would agree it is sadly missing in our present hospital system. Patient-centered design allows for visual and acoustical privacy, as well as opportunities for social contact. For example, Wright (1992) describes the experience of one patient with cancer who desperately needed someone to talk to about his fears and his concerns for his family. When the social worker finally arrived, she pulled the curtain around his bed, separating him from his roommate. After the visit, the social worker left thinking how well the patient was adjusting to his cancer. In the meantime, the man silently wept. There was no way he could talk about his fears with his roommate listening. St. Charles Medical Center in Bend, Oregon, is addressing this need by adding a private consultation room on their oncology unit.

At the same time, social isolation is a stressor that may heighten sensitivity to pain and slow healing (Speedling and Rosenberg, 1986). Providing comfortable lounges where patients can talk among themselves and visit with families can lessen this stress. At Planetree, staff members find that patients are the best teachers and support for other patients. No one knows as well as other patients how it feels to have an illness or to go through a surgery (Gilpin and Nelson, 1991).

Symbolic Meaning. The physical environment conveys meaning. A patient-centered environment that focuses on the psychosocial needs of patients will be considered caring and positive, while an environment that focuses primarily on providers sends a negative message and makes patients and visitors feel unimportant (Carpman, Grant, and Simmons, 1986). For example, consider the message conveyed to a patient lying on a stretcher with harsh florescent light glaring from above. Now, consider the message when there is a serene nature-scene poster on the ceiling and soft music playing in the background.

Promoting Patient Control

As we mentioned earlier, the patient's sense of being in control is a well-documented contribution to a rapid healing process.

Designs that reduce stress and empower patients offer opportunities for them to participate actively in controlling their environment — for example, by being able to control their television, lights, and room temperature. Baier (1989) reminds us how important temperature control is for the very ill. "Often I mentioned being too warm. I was told, however, there were many elderly people with poor circulation in the unit and I would just have to accept the situation" (p. 15). Planetree allows patients access to food as a way of providing a sense of control. Patients can go to the kitchen and get something to eat anytime during night or day. In a traditional system patients are dependent on others to bring food to them. Also, Planetree has a nutritionist who provides information as she helps patients prepare food.

Creating a Homelike Atmosphere

The institutionalized design of traditional hospitals is perceived as intimidating and disempowering by the very population it is intended to serve. When environments seem familiar and homelike, patients are likely to feel relaxed and to take part in health-producing activities, such as walking. Patients who are more active have fewer complications such as pneumonia and blood clots than patients who are not active.

Healing Through the Physical Senses

An environment that appeals to the senses is an important component of the healing process. For example, research supports the intuitive sense that access to nature aids healing. Ulrich (1991) found that the environmental factors most effective in reducing stress and enhancing wellness have been the same throughout the ages. These factors include natural elements, such as trees, plants, water, and animals, and happy faces and artwork that represents serene nature scenes. During a study of the effects of various ceiling-mounted pictures, Cross (1990) found that patients exposed to serene pictures, such as pastoral scenes, had lower blood pressure than those exposed to arousing pictures (sailboarders or animals looking at observers) or than those who had no pictures.

Another example of the role of the senses in healing is the effects of the smell of baking breads and homemade soups from Planetree's kitchen. As one observer said, "The hospital didn't smell like a hospital anymore. The kitchen becomes a wonderful place to be when this occurs, prompting visits from other people throughout the hospital" (Gilpin and Nelson, 1991, p. 147). Also, some hospitals are using aroma therapy to help patients relax. For example, the use of the vanilla fragrance has been effective in helping patients relax during magnetic resonance scans.

The most frequent complaint I hear from patients is about noise. Noise comes from all over: talking in the halls, equipment being moved, doors banging, other patients' televisions blaring, and the incessant paging. It seems ironic that being able to rest peacefully in the hospital is the exception rather than the norm. As we have mentioned earlier, relaxation and rest are essential components of a healing environment. Patient-centered care challenges hospitals to find ways to meet this important consumer need through the use of technology and by restructuring processes. For example, the use of vibrating beepers for locating staff can eliminate the need for overhead paging, and cross-training staff can decrease the number of people interacting with patients. In addition, music and fountains may be used to soften the acoustical environment.

Facilitating Healing

In summary, it is important to include healing in health care because the needs of the whole person are the focus of care. The focus must be on the person and the underlying causes contributing to the illness because the more we can identify underlying causes and help patients and their family become active participants in their health, the less likely it is that problems will recur or persist.

Furthermore, Kaiser (1992) reminds us that our presence with patients is just as important as what we do with them. With a patient-focused approach conversations with patients are intentional; they enable, inspire, and educate. Kaiser offers a useful metaphor: the hospital is a university. Patients and their families should come through the hospital experience knowing more than they did when they went in. They are empowered through having information, making their own decisions, and practicing the skills they need for continued healing and recovery. Among these skills are mind/body therapies, proven to facilitate healing, which patients and families can learn to do for themselves and continue using after hospitalization.

As a result, patient-focused care makes good economic sense, for all these methods contribute to increased patient satisfaction, shorter lengths of stay, and less need for readmission because of complications. All these are important economic incentives for hospitals given DRG reimbursement, managed care, and an increasingly competitive environment.

A patient-centered model of care recognizes that everything in the hospital experience contributes to patient healing. In Chapter Five we explore this healing environment further as we examine how its creation affects the health care team.

Chapter 4

Restructuring Hospitals for Patient-Focused Care

> Throughout nature, growth involves periodic accelerations and
> transformations: Things go slowly for a time and nothing
> seems to change—until suddenly the eggshell cracks, the
> branch blossoms, the tadpole's tail shrinks away, the leaf falls,
> the bird molts, the hibernation begins. With us it is the same.
>
> William Bridges, *Transitions**

Restructuring is not for the timid. It is a major undertaking that reaches across the breadth and into the depths of
the organization. It requires a bird's-eye view of the work of
the organization. It also requires that the information gained
be used in an unbiased and objective way. Many organizational
members will need to expand or redefine the roles they have
grown comfortable with, and some may no longer be needed.
Restructuring must be carefully managed so that everyone is
included in helping create the change.

In this chapter, we present strategies and options for restructuring hospitals for patient-focused care. We answer the
question of how to begin by exploring the importance of assessing the unique characteristics and requirements of each setting.
Then we explore the role of consultants in the process and outline general guiding principles and steps for implementation.
In order to facilitate understanding of implementation, we present examples from a few hospitals that have been through the

*William Bridges, *Transitions: Making Sense of Life's Changes,* ©1980 by
Addison-Wesley Publishing Co. Reprinted by permission of Addison-Wesley Publishing Co., Inc., Reading, Mass.

process. We next address management of the emotional side
of the change process. We close this chapter with a review of
the problems and lessons learned.

Where to Begin?

Hospitals come in all sizes and stages of development. Yet they all
share one main characteristic: they are one of the most complex
organizations of our time. Peter Drucker informs us, "You [health
care] are not the toy industry. You are deeply involved in the
public interest. We expect more from the healthcare system than
from the toy industry. Ten or 15 years ago there was tremendous satisfaction with the American healthcare system. . . .
Today there is enormous dissatisfaction" (quoted in Flower,
1991, p. 58).

It is no longer a question of whether to change; it is only
a question of choosing the kind of change. In order for a hospital to become patient-focused by improving service and quality
while reducing costs, it is important to begin with an analysis
of the unique characteristics and requirements of the organization. Questions that need to be answered in this analysis are:

> What is the hospital's present financial position?
> What is its operational efficiency?
> What are the internal resources for promoting change,
>   such as analytical and facilitation expertise?
> What are the staff and management capabilities?
> What have been the previous experiences with internal
>   initiatives for change?
> How urgently is the need for change perceived by orga-
>   nizational members?
> How likely is the organization to sustain current success?
> How strong is the motivation to be an industry leader?
> Do all groups in the hospital share a common vision?
> Who are the formal and informal leaders?

When most hospitals begin pondering these questions, they turn
to consultants.

Role of Consultants

Few organizations have the people, time, expertise, or energy to perform the rigorous work of structural change. Even when they do, they often find they are much like fish, which, Einstein said, "will be the last to discover water" (cited by Kurtz, 1990, p. 17). This inability to see the forest for the trees is a characteristic of human nature and is based on how the mind works. When information is transmitted to the mind, it is connected to constructs, or cognitive maps of how things and people function. These cognitive maps develop as a result of formal learning, vicarious experiences, and direct experiences. Some maps we are actively aware of, and others are in the background of our awareness. They are significant in that they help organize and give meaning to material. Yet, at the same time, they act as filters and distorters of information. The information that filters through tends to be that which is consistent with existing cognitive maps. Utilizing outside consultants to facilitate transformation helps organizations broaden their vision by considering information that is inconsistent with their cognitive maps. Opening to new possibilities in this way is a key to implementing patient-focused care because throughout the process there is a natural tendency for departments, professions, and the organization itself to defend boundaries and the usual way of operating.

Hospitals need to identify the unique needs they want consultants to fulfill before choosing consultants because in the final analysis success will depend on the commitment of the organization itself. Saint Joseph's Hospital of Atlanta, for example, chose to utilize consultants only during the initial phase of their restructuring process, as they had sufficient internal expertise for implementation. At Saint Joseph's, the consultants worked intensively with the project team for about six weeks, providing education and initial data. According to chief executive officer Jim Lussier, St. Charles Medical Center, a 180-bed rural referral center located in Bend, Oregon, based their choice of consultants on a desire for good analytical and facilitation skills. One of the major goals of St. Charles was to develop a process that could be followed by their own staff, who were trained to continue the process after the consultants left.

The following are some general guidelines (Distasio, 1988; Scheuerman and Smith, 1992) for deciding when to use consultants and determining how to choose them.

Consultants should be used when any of the following conditions are present:

1. The organization lacks qualified persons who can initiate, oversee, or follow through with the project.
2. The organization has qualified persons, but they lack the time, energy, or resources to accomplish the project.
3. The internal restructuring is on a large scale, causing anxiety and resistance and the need for an external, unbiased perspective.
4. The organization has a close deadline for completion of the process and internal resources cannot accomplish it within the compressed time frame.

The following factors need to be considered when choosing consultants:

1. The scope of the project—for example, the number of departments affected, how multidisciplinary personnel will be affected, the anticipated time frame, the reporting and accountability lines that need to be established.
2. Whether a canned or customized design approach is desired. Canned programs require the organization to fit into a prepackaged system. At this point in the development of patient-focused care, an approach that is customized to the unique needs of the particular organization is probably desirable.
3. The flexibility of the system suggested. In today's environment of rapid change any system consultants recommend must be flexible and easy to modify.
4. The creativity and clarity of the consultant's approach. One way creativity and clarity can be assessed is by providing consultants with general guidelines, including the purpose

of the project, goals and objectives, and time frames, and evaluating how they translate these general guidelines into the specifics of the project.

5.   The roles and responsibilities of the consultants. The consultants' role should be based on the needs of the organization. For example, will they function as educators and trainers? Will they be expected to manage the human side of implementation as well as the analytical side? Will they be responsible for monitoring and follow-up and for how long?

6.   The qualifications and expertise of the consultants. For example, what are their educational background and previous experience with patient-focused restructuring? In addition, how long have they worked together as a team? What is their track record for giving personalized, customized service as assessed through references?

7.   The consultants' fit to the organization's culture. For example, do the consultants show an interest in and sensitivity to the organization's culture? Also, how compatible are the consultants' personalities and the organization's culture?

8.   The cost. In evaluating cost, both the cost of using consultants and the cost of not doing so need to be considered. Reputable consulting firms will have a fair, reasonable cost quotation. According to Distasio (1988, p. 10), "If a project cost seems too good to be true — that is, inexpensive in relation to the scope of the project — it is. The old adage, 'you get what you pay for' holds true when purchasing consultive services." Among the ways to reduce costs are to seek grants, assign some tasks to in-house staff, break the project down into phases or stages, and fund each stage separately.

Guiding Principles

For patient-focused care to succeed, the culture of the organization must shift from the traditional provider focus to a patient focus. Three principles must be used to guide the process: systems thinking, the active participation of staff, and visionary leadership.

Systems Thinking

Systems thinking involves a shift away from the analytical, mechanical, one-way, causal thinking of classical science toward examination of a whole process and of the interrelationship of the great number of variables that constitute the process. The rigorous application of systems thinking is rare. Although systems thinking is quite natural in children, most of us have been trained since childhood to think in analytical ways, to "confront our problems in a spirit of divide-and-conquer. Consequently, systems thinking requires that we pay attention to habits of thought that we ordinarily take for granted" (Davidson, 1983, p. 30).

Davidson (1983, p. 31) offers a simple exercise that he uses in his university course on problem solving to demonstrate systems thinking. He offers his students this code to break:

MZQPQ LPQ AZQ XUCMX CT FQXAQPFQLP?

If you are having difficulty, you are probably looking at the parts instead of the whole. You are probably looking at individual words or letters instead of the whole sentence. Viewing it as a whole, the first thing you notice is that it is a question. "In as much as questions commonly begin with words like WHO, WHAT, WHEN, WHERE, and, WHY, you can guess that the first word, being five letters, is WHERE. Now, go for the soft spots of the system. Try the second and third words rather than the ten-letter monster at the end. If the first word is WHERE, the next two words must end with RE and HE, as in ARE and THE." Eureka, you now have enough letters to determine the complete message through a trial and error process in which you eliminate unlikely words. Here is the message (from "The Ballad of Women of Olden Times" by François Villon):

WHERE ARE THE SNOWS OF YESTERYEAR?

This code is unsolvable by focusing simply on its parts. The solution begins to emerge when one focuses on the whole and on the way the individual parts relate to one another to form the whole. This is the heart of systems thinking. This perspective avoids a common pitfall of problem solving: the tendency to concentrate on an isolated part of the problem rather than on the whole picture. This limited perspective blocks the resolution of many problems that reoccur time and time again because their root cause has never been addressed. Systems thinking assists in making patterns clear and therefore allows us to see how to change these patterns effectively.

Systems thinking applies the concept of structure to explain the conflict between behavior and values. In systems thinking, structure is the key interrelationships that generate specific, compelling patterns of behavior. Nearly everyone in health care will say the patient is the focus of care, yet because the structure of the system they are in focuses more on their department or profession than on the patient, they are precluded from functioning effectively as part of a truly patient-focused-care team. For example, when management engineers entered hospitals to study processes, they found that 20 percent of the wage dollar goes to structured idle time (Lathrop, 1991) as a direct result of the hospital structure and operating approach.

In order to change the structure it is important first to understand that structure by obtaining hard data through rigorous analysis. Changes must be based on data, not on personal opinions, exaggeration, and mistaken understandings. The importance of this guiding principle cannot be overstated. Deming, credited with transforming Japanese industry and a modern-day guru for TQM, points out that applying statistical methods is essential for minimizing confusion and for the positive transformation of American business: "In God we trust. All others must use data" (cited by Walton, 1986, p. 96). Furthermore, he says, "Statistical methods help to understand processes, to bring them under control, and then to improve them. Otherwise, people will forever be 'putting out fires' rather than improving the system" (p. 96).

For restructuring, Henderson and Williams (1991b) recommend that the analysis focus on operational issues — such as patient mix, operating methods, census patterns, and acuity levels—and on personnel issues including work fit, work issues, organizational climate, policies and procedures, and work-site involvement. Yet, as Deming points out, data without context or inaccurate data may be harmful (Walton, 1986). It is necessary to know the context and nature of the data and to ensure that proper data are utilized as well.

The most useful statistical tools are neither complicated nor difficult to master. Many of these tools are merely ways of visually displaying and organizing data in a meaningful way. Most often, employees can be empowered through education to collect and interpret this data on their own. Some of the tools staff can learn to use include cause-and-effect diagrams, flow charts, pareto charts, run (trend) charts, histograms, control charts, and scatter diagrams. An in-depth explanation of these tools is beyond the scope of this book. We refer the reader to the many books now available on TQM.

Active Staff Participation

Staff involvement and participation are equally as important as accurate data and rigorous analysis. In general, people do not resist change, they resist being changed. It is important to empower employees because they are closest to the customer and have a great deal of knowledge of customer needs. Given the opportunity, employees have many ideas for improving quality and reducing cost. Henderson and Williams (1991a) offer an 80–20 rule to guide planning. In order for the process to have staff buy-in, only 20 percent of the analysis should be from the top down. A full 80 percent of the effort should be through participative analysis, decisions, and implementation. "Spend a majority of the time gathering input and data from staff, analyzing and interpreting the data with the staff, deciding on the best course of action, and implementing the plan with full staff participation" (p. 50).

For example, Gomberg and Miller (1992, p. 71) identified organizational focus and commitment as the main factors in the restructuring effort at Lee Memorial Medical Center, 627 beds housed in two campuses in Fort Myers, Florida. They found that staff involvement in creating the new delivery model fostered commitment, trust, enthusiasm, and ownership of the success. In addition, it set in place the process and structure to empower staff at the patient-contact level.

Visionary Leadership

The commitment to patient-focused care must begin at the top and filter through every level, every department, and every individual in the hospital. The patient-focused approach requires placing the patient and family at the center and creating a partnership of physicians, nurses, and all hospital staff to care for and serve the patient. The direction for this process begins with the CEO.

Each of the hospitals launching patient-focused efforts is led by a visionary CEO who is willing to take the risk to change the organization and usher in a new era. Embarking on this process requires courage, vision, and faith. It means virtually reinventing the hospital by transforming policies, practices, and the physical environment. Leadership during a change process of this magnitude is very risky, and, as one CEO states, "Leaders must be ready to take some flack, spend some money, and get some resistance" (quoted in Weber, 1991, p. 23). As the organizational hierarchy and departmental barriers are challenged, leadership must be empowered with information and committed to the change. They must have a strong commitment to the overall success of the entire organization in order not to cave in to the pressures of special interests. Leaders must gaze into the future and visualize the challenges, risks, and opportunities that lie ahead.

Hospitals that have undertaken patient-focused restructuring describe it as a sea change. It requires a willingness to invest a great deal of money, time, and energy in order to achieve long-term gains. It also requires a willingness to make mistakes. Leaders who have implemented patient-focused care had a vision of the ultimate end product, despite the fact that they did not have written long-range strategic plans. It seems to be a journey of discovery rather than of following a set plan. Because patient-focused restructuring is still experimental, and all the models now being implemented are still being evaluated, it is important to prepare individuals for handling the inevitable mistakes and problems that will occur. It is important for top leadership to nurture the mind-set that views mistakes as providing information helpful for learning rather than as failures. The driving force that inspired these leaders was the belief that in the long run this approach would result in significant quality improvements, increased customer satisfaction, increased market share, and decreased labor cost.

Unfortunately, the type of high-performance teamwork needed for this effort is not usually evidenced at the top management and leadership levels. According to Sibbet and O'Hara-Devereaux, "These major stake holders have held individual — often competing — visions. . . . Lacking a shared vision, [they] frequently travel through the same territory in isolation from each other. When the organization hits turbulent times, they don't have common directional tools to maintain organizational stability and direction" (1991, p. 27). Top management will not work as a team of its own accord without conscious attention to group process and creating a common vision and framework that can be understood and shared by all. Once top management is working together, the message must be reinforced by all management staff because they are the leaders for their departments. All managers must communicate the vision and value of patient-focused care and reward appropriate employee behavior and attitudes.

Because vision is central to the success of any change process and to achieving goals, it may be helpful to review the concept of vision and how leaders can use the power of vision to create commitment for a successful change process. A vision is a vivid visual image of a desired future for an organization. For our purpose, it is a description of how the unit or entire hospital will function once patient-focused care is in place. The vision should include how patients will be treated, how ancillary services will be provided, how caregivers' roles will change, how teams of cross-trained individuals will interact, and any other elements of patient-focused care. The more detailed the

6. Involve cross-functional teams in solving problems and designing systems.
7. Reward behaviors consistent with teamwork and patient-focused care.
8. Be clear about the reasons for implementing patient-focused care.
9. Anticipate mistakes and problems and define them as opportunities for learning.
10. Concentrate on the positive and express confidence in the future.

Steps in the Transformation Process

The transformation process involves constantly challenging assumptions and the status quo. Throughout the process, people are challenged to forget the present system and think about their patients, answering the following questions: What are the needs of a particular group of patients? Are patients grouped according to need? Based on patient needs, what are the services and resources that belong on a particular unit? What is the best way to allocate these resources to the patient-care area?

David Bellaire and George Sauter (1992) summarize this strategy in process engineering terms: simply put, the challenge for hospitals today is to efficiently and effectively match resources to demand. According to Bellaire and Sauter this strategy involves:

1. *Defining the dimensions of demand (patients).*
   What is the present demand?
   How predictable is the demand?
   How is the supply (staff, services, technology) currently matched to demand?
2. *Deciding how to reconfigure demand.*
   Is there a better way to aggregate patients?
   Is there a better way to schedule admissions or surgeries (or both)?
3. *Determining the best way to allocate resources to the newly configured patient-care areas.*
   Move services to the patient when this change is affordable.

Simplify processes and tasks.

Eliminate non-value-added activities.

Expand case management.

Use exception-based, protocol-driven charting.

Leverage highly skilled professionals (that is, use highly skilled professionals' talents in the most cost-effective way by using less-skilled staff to perform more routine tasks).

Streamline decision making and flatten the management structure.

Consolidate volume-sensitive services (that is, low- or variable-usage services such as EKG, EEG, ultrasound, and x-ray).

In addition, APM consultant Bellaire identifies five elements key to the success of major organizational change initiatives:

1. The change process must be driven by an operating vision and a set of specific, measurable targets.

2. The change must occur within a disciplined time frame. The change process must have enough momentum to overcome inertia toward changing the old system.

3. The change must seem significant to leadership. Leadership is unlikely to maintain interest in any change unless it is seen as having an overall impact on the organization. For example, the goal of getting hot food to patients alone may not be enough to sustain leadership interest even though it is a worthy goal. Grouping initiatives according to cost and quality outcomes will make it more likely that these goals receive support and focus.

4. Just-in-time training must be used. If new tools are learned too far in advance of their application, they will likely be forgotten. Training at the time of need ensures increased success.

5. A set of measurement and management tools to sustain the new behaviors and culture must be adopted. Without proper measurement tools and ongoing data to assess success in achieving goals and targets, the change process will falter.

In implementing this strategy, it helps to have a map. At the same time, it is wise to remember that the map is not the territory. Each organization will need to adapt the map to its unique needs and culture. And, much like the explorers of new lands, participants in patient-focused restructuring will discover unforeseen obstacles and need to reroute their path. Sometimes they will repeat previous steps or refine a process or skill.

Before beginning the journey, it is important to lay the foundation, which consists of convincing the organization of the need for change and assuring that the change is in line with the mission and values of the organization. For example, St. Charles Medical Center began laying the foundation a full year prior to restructuring with the disclosure of the hospital's financial status including projections for the future. Fortunately, as with all the hospitals now involved in patient-focused restructuring, the hospital was in a stable financial position, but projections into the future under present operating methods indicated a shrinking margin with a budget deficit within three years. Bellaire graphically explains the problem. "The capacity to create revenues within the constraints of managed care are practically nonexistent. Therefore, the focus for strategies [lies] in reducing cost through greater operational efficiency" (personal communication).

Henderson and Williams of the Hay Group (1991a, pp. 50–53) offer a useful map, summarizing the change process in ten practical steps.

1. Identify and communicate the vision, goals, and process.
2. Assess current data, identifying gaps and developing plans for gathering new data.
3. Identify pilot units based on their overall readiness, need for improvement, and management capability and support.
4. Involve staff in planning.
5. Collect and analyze additional data as necessary.
6. Discuss findings, obtaining feedback before developing conclusions.
7. Develop a plan for change that emphasizes the reallocation and flow of work tasks.

8. Develop detailed recommendations, action plans, and time
    tables through group participation.
9. Review each unit's plan with top management, who in turn
    will assess the plan in the light of the original objectives
    and criteria.
10. Implement the plan and evaluate it. "In actual practice,
    steps 5 through 10 may be repeated at a number of levels.
    With each new level, diagnosis becomes more focused, ac-
    tion plans become more specific and solutions become
    more accepted."

In the second step, data gathering can be organized into
two basic areas — operations and staff, physician, and patient perceptions. External operations analyses include comparisons with
other similar and reputable hospitals. Internal factors that need
to be analyzed include skill mix, bed utilization, transfer rates,
operating-room utilization, scheduling, census by patient unit,
average admissions by day and by patient type, and the following:

- Work flow, or the relationship and sequencing of work steps
  in a process: Analyzing work flow exposes inefficiency, redundancy, and misunderstanding.
- Time utilization and work sampling: The goal of work sampling is to break the labor hour into components that describe
  how time is being spent.
- Work loads — the turnaround times and quantity of work
  required for services.
- Existing and desired models of care delivery — primary care,
  team nursing, or case management.
- Physical environment: How does the physical environment
  support patient-focused care? What are the constraints and
  opportunities for improvement?
- Technology utilization: What are the present technologies?
  What is the skill level needed to use them? What is the impact of current and anticipated automation on staffing?
- Organizational structure: How is work allocated throughout the organization? Is it focused on the customer? What
  is the hierarchy? How does communication flow? How are

responsibility and accountability aligned? What oversight is needed to assure effective patient-focused care?

- Future plans: What are the plans for equipment, facilities, or services that affect staffing and customer service?
- Certification, licensing, and accreditation implications: How does professional licensing and certification constrain cross-training and the development of multiskilled workers? What are the implications of standards from accrediting agencies?

Analyzing staff, physician, and patient perceptions includes reviewing previous satisfaction surveys and meeting minutes to identify concerns, as well as conducting focus groups, interviews, and surveys. The process includes gathering information in order to answer these questions:

How satisfied are these groups with the present system?
What problems and issues do they identify?
What ideas do they have for improvement?
What are their expectations?

Successful Transformations

Now we will look at how various hospitals have successfully implemented patient-focused restructuring.

Lakeland Regional Medical Center

At the forefront of these pioneering hospitals is Lakeland Regional Medical Center, an 897-bed hospital in Lakeland, Florida (Weber, 1991). In 1987 Lakeland management became convinced that "preservation of the status quo was clearly going to lead us into a tragic crisis situation" (p. 24). With the help of consultants, managers began the rigorous research and analysis necessary to begin restructuring. By 1989 the pilot was ready to begin. A forty-bed surgical unit was transformed into a self-contained surgical service with its own minilaboratory, diagnostic radiology rooms, administrative records/clerical area, and supply stockrooms.

To facilitate this transformation, several key changes were made. First, the managers charted the steps and amount of actual utilization of each job. Then, they identified work duplication and how much time each service actually spent in care delivery. As a result, services previously not located on the unit were moved to the patient care area when this was found to be cost-effective. They eliminated the nurses' station, creating in its place a central area for offices surrounded by a pharmacy and other services that the staff could access easily.

The next key change was the creation of multiskilled practitioners. After an intensive six weeks of training and successful completion of competency tests, these practitioners were prepared to take care of 90 percent of their patient's needs, including providing limited respiratory therapy, providing basic physical therapy, doing EKGs, organizing schedules, performing phlebotomy and laboratory tests, charging and charting at bedside computers, keeping medical records, providing transportation, setting diets, cleaning up rooms, performing minor engineering services, and doing a variety of tasks that do not fit in traditional job descriptions. These multiskilled practitioners were organized into "care pairs" (Loudin, 1991, p. 8) consisting of an RN and another health care worker. The care pairs follow their four to seven patients from preadmission to discharge. Preadmission and precertification were located on the floor, allowing care pairs to meet with their patients prior to admission. According to Phyllis Watson, vice-president of nursing, one of the driving concepts is to "do more and more things for fewer people" (quoted in Weber, 1991, p. 25). As a result, these multiskilled workers truly provide continuity in care.

Another key change was providing consistency of care across all shifts. The care pairs care for the same physician's patients to provide continuity. When a physician calls the master scheduler to schedule a surgery, the master scheduler links the physician's office with the operating room via a conference call. At this time the physician can choose whether she wants to schedule the patient so that she works with her primary team or, because of time constraints, with her secondary team. Immediately, the patient is tied into the work load of the appropriate care pairs covering all three shifts.

In addition to these key changes, Watson identifies five other changes that enabled the transformation to succeed: charting-by-exception, introduction of computer systems, provision for compensation and career advancement, implementation of a silent communication system, and cross-training. Charting-by-exception involves the use of flow sheets, five-day records on which all caregivers, including physicians, document their care. Protocols for care are used, and only exceptions to the anticipated recovery process are documented. According to Watson, one no longer sees such superfluous notes as "skin warm and dry, patient sleeping." One example of a patient-focused activity included in the protocol is for the caregiver to sit down with the patient between 6 P.M. and 10 P.M. every evening to review how the patient is progressing. This time is greatly appreciated by patients. They learn how they are progressing relative to the standard protocol and what they can expect throughout the rest of their stay. They also have an opportunity to ask questions and learn why certain treatments are being performed.

Another change was the initiation of a housewide computer information system, which includes master scheduling, bedside charting, charging, and admissions, transfer, and discharge information.

The career-advancement system rewards flexibility as achieved through education, competency testing, licensing, and professional development. The system has two parts. Part A assesses skills through competency testing, educational level, and licensing. Each of these areas is given predetermined points and the pay scale is adjusted accordingly. Part B is modeled after the nursing clinical ladder system and rewards multiskilled workers with pay differentials in conjunction with continued professional development.

The silent communication system has done a great deal for continuity of care. The surgical service has only one phone, which is answered by the receptionist. Messages for caregivers are transmitted via vibrating alphanumeric pagers. Caregivers receive their messages silently without being interrupted in their patient care. They take note of each message and, if necessary, can respond via one of the strategically located zone phones.

An excellent plan for cross-training prepared employees for their new multiskilled roles. For the six-week training period, the education department and various clinical specialists developed modular programs. They used a variety of teaching methods including classroom instruction, videos, touch-screen interactive computers, laboratory simulations, and clinical experience. These sessions were followed with competency training and evaluation. In addition, Watson emphasizes the importance of team building. The team-building process focused on developing multidisciplinary teams and furthering the overall vision for the project.

Dennis Shortridge, executive vice-president and chief operating officer of Lakeland, says restructuring is a never-ending process. "We continually learn from the implementation of each unit and have not found a universal method for restructuring. . . . We will continue to learn from our experiences during the next few years and will revisit past units to make improvements" (Sasenick, 1992b). Lakeland now has a plan for creating five operating units, or minihospitals, which will involve the entire medical center in the restructuring.

St. Charles Medical Center

"Forget this hospital exists. Imagine that nothing is here. Think about your patients and their needs. How would you design your unit to meet those needs?" said Rick Martin, vice president of operations of St. Charles Medical Center in Bend, Oregon, when St. Charles committed to hospitalwide restructuring of all departments and services in January 1992. This restructuring is unique because St. Charles integrated healing health care principles, which focus on enhancing the healing environment. Here are the principles (adapted version):

Principle	*Example*
Respect the dignity, rights, and contributions of employees.	Involve employees and physicians in operations redesign.

Move services to patients.

Reconfigure patient units to reduce costs and improve quality.

Make the most out of clinical experts.

Balance work and redesign jobs.

Align authority, responsibility, and outcomes.

Consolidate low or variable volume services.

Define best practice.

Improve efficiency and simplify work.

Flatten management structure.

Combine art and science of medicine.

Enhance the healing environment.

Decentralize ancillary, adminstrative, and support services to units.

Cluster "like" patients on units and operate at full capacity whenever possible.

Restructure and/or eliminate daily tasks.

Cross-train personnel so that they are multiskilled.

Consolidate services and responsibility on patient units and give units increased accountability for outcomes.

Centralize expensive, immovable equipment.

Expand case management and critical paths (that is, standardized, daily plans for care).

Eliminate waste and reduce redundancy.

Reduce management layers and streamline decision making.

Increase involvement of patient and family. Meet physical, emotional, social, intellectual, and spiritual needs.

Provide more homelike atmosphere. Improve knowledge and methods.

These principles served as guidelines for each unit as it created patient-centered designs. Each unit differentiated its approach based on the unique needs of its specific patient population. For example, the orthopedic unit created a focus team consisting of unit-based physical therapists, occupational therapists, nurses, multiskilled workers called "care associates," a nursing case manager, supply technicians, a unit secretary, and a unit manager. In addition, designated social services personnel and pharmacists work consistently with the team, although they still report to their respective department managers.

Devising a Plan for Transformation. St. Charles, under the guidance of consultants, used a process with four phases: setup, strategy development, design, and implementation. The setup phase included setting the overall direction and ground rules, organizing the project, developing a general human resource plan, developing a communication plan, identifying education and learning needs, and gathering data and analyzing.

The overall direction was planned by senior management. The outcome of their effort was a well-articulated vision, goals, and guiding principles for the process. This first step was crucial for the success of the entire process. The vision, goals, and principles were a vital part of keeping the process on track and moving toward the targets. When clearly and repeatedly articulated, such principles help reduce the natural anxieties people have during change because they know why the changes are necessary and where the organization is heading.

Organizing the project involved developing an overall structure and an efficient reporting process. This part of the setup phase was the backbone of the process because it was based on the unique culture of the organization. St. Charles organized the project by establishing a project team, a steering committee, an operating team, and task forces. The project team, consisting of both consultants and hospital personnel, provided overall support. Its role was to do the behind-the-scenes work of developing and analyzing data and the up-front work of facilitating the process. In addition, it developed hypotheses for change that served as guidelines for the work of both the steering committee and the task forces.

In addition, a steering committee guided the process and provided direction. This committee consisted of representatives of senior management, physicians, and staff members. The various task forces and the operating team reported the results of their work to the steering committee. The steering committee set cost and service targets, approved strategies, reviewed progress, approved operational design ideas, and oversaw implementation.

The operating team was a short-term group consisting of middle managers. This team developed the overall operating strategy, then dissolved into task forces. Many of the operating team members became chairpersons of the task forces, which were charged with designing the patient-focused-care units. They consisted of representatives of the nurses, ancillary-service personnel, support staff, physicians, and other groups involved in meeting the needs of patients. They were guided by the restructuring principles and the cost and service targets set by the steering committee. Project-team members acted as facilitators and supported the process by providing relevant data.

Early in any restructuring process it is important to have a general human relations policy statement regarding people who will be displaced because of changes. This issue must be dealt with in an honest, forthright manner at the beginning of the process. The critical questions are "Will there be layoffs?" and "How will those who are displaced be utilized?"

St. Charles created a transition team to handle these issues. Based on the restructuring principles and the stable financial position of the hospital, it chose a no-layoff policy according to which every attempt was made to find creative and meaningful work for all displaced workers until natural attrition of 20 percent per year created vacancies. The transition team instituted a freeze on filling positions and created a job-storage program. Each request to fill a position was evaluated individually. Some positions were filled if they required narrowly defined expertise; some were filled on a temporary basis; and some needs were met through cross-training or retraining existing staff. The plan was to use displaced staff in creative ways, such as having them mentor staff members who were moving into new roles, provide health-related community services, and complete specific projects. The staff members for newly created positions were recruited internally, and the hospital paid for the additional training required. This process was welcomed by many who now had new career opportunities. For example, some of the new care associates were previously phlebotomists who wanted increased patient contact and the opportunity to learn new skills; others were environmental-services personnel who wanted eventually to become nurses.

At the same time, a communications plan was developed that answered certain questions: Who needs to know about the restructuring? What does each group need to know? How is the information best communicated? Those who needed to know included managers, supervisors, staff, physicians, and the community. Hospitals that have been through this process emphasize that "you can't communicate enough" and "when you think you have communicated all you can, communicate some more." What was communicated depended on the audience. Physicians, for example, needed to understand what they would gain from the changes, how care for their patients would improve, how bureaucracy would decrease, how communication would improve, and how information for decision making would flow. Managers and supervisors are keys to successful communication efforts. They set the tone for their departments; however, middle management is often the group that has the most at stake in maintaining the present culture. Efforts to inform managers fully and to set clear standards and articulate a clear vision will pay off many times over.

Every effort was made to keep staff fully informed. Inherent in the restructuring process, as in any major change process, are anxiety and fear and the rumors that often follow. A variety of communication methods was used including town meetings, rap sessions, department meetings, voice mail, computer networks, newsletters, posters, notebooks with task-force meeting minutes, and roving project team members.

Early in the process, St. Charles released a press statement to the community explaining the purpose of the process and the overall goals of cost reduction and service enhancement. This strategy helped dispel the inevitable rumors engendered by the anxiety accompanying the change process.

How the community will be informed needs to be thoroughly examined. Hospitals that have been through the process recommend planning press conferences. Also, it is beneficial to release, early in the process, a press statement explaining the purpose of the process and the overall goals of cost reduction and service enhancement.

At the beginning of the process, St. Charles identified learning needs and developed educational programs. The skills that needed to be taught included data gathering and analysis as well as how to conduct successful meetings. In addition, St. Charles and its community college developed educational programs for new positions such as the multiskilled ones utilized in patient-focused care.

The second phase was strategy development. After an initial analysis was completed, as described previously in this chapter, operating challenges were identified. Like other hospitals that have reorganized, St. Charles Medical Center identified a high variability in day-to-day work load, high within-day workload variability, and temporary capacity crises, which led to incorrect patient placement on care units. In short, all the patient units were constantly needing to adjust to a seemingly unpredictable work load. The implications included:

- A cost of nearly $400,000 per year because of the inability to adjust staffing quickly enough to the wide variation in patient census.
- Physician dissatisfaction because less experienced and less specialized nurses were caring for their patients.
- Staff dissatisfaction related to lack of knowledge and expertise in caring for specialized patients; frequent shortages and the calling off of regular staff related to unmanaged demand.
- Wasted resources as a result of patient transfers.
- The need for a rich skill mix, which meant staffing mostly with RNs, and high nursing hours per patient day. The cost was nearly $350,000 per year.
- Inconsistent and fragmented delivery of patient care with an average of thirty-five different people involved in a patient's care during a four-day hospital stay.
- Only 24 percent of an RN's time going to actual patient care.
- An inability to develop case management and to deliver the best care and service possible.

After analyzing and discussing the data, the operating team chose a focus care design on each patient unit. Four key themes drove the focus care design: demand management, job redesign, decentralization, and scheduling. The demand strategy was to divide each unit into focus and flex areas. In the focus area, patients were grouped by using DRGs to predict similar needs. Such grouping ensured high occupancy in this area of the unit. The flex area received patients who were more unpredictable in their needs, such as emergency patients. As a result, the census in the flex area was more variable. Job redesign consisted of redefining job criteria and skill mix to optimize the use of scarce or expensive resources, such as RNs, to increase team members' flexibility, and to reduce nonpatient care activities, such as documentation. Because the same grouping of patients is always in the focus area, the team gets to know their care regime in depth and is able to concentrate on performing with excellence. An added bonus is that team members know their schedules and therefore are not constantly being asked to go home or come in according to the previous variability in patient census. As the patient population becomes more predictable, it will be possible to even out the staff mix to make a multi-skilled team that utilizes care associates, instead of having units almost entirely comprised of RNs. Decentralization means bringing services to the patient, whenever it is cost-effective, and reducing low-value-added activities, such as documentation and the transporting of patients to and from other departments. Scheduling is key to success for focused care on surgical units. As the patient care units planned their design, the director of surgical services began the process of working with physicians to align the surgery schedule with overall patient care needs through using master scheduling systems and case management to better forecast, plan, and schedule.

Once patients were grouped according to needs and predictability, the services they require were studied. When the utilization of a service such as physical therapy, social services, or occupational therapy was high enough to make it cost-effective, it could be permanently included on the unit. For example, patients of the orthopedic focus team required at least eight hours a day of both occupational and physical therapy; as a result, a physical therapist and an occupational therapist were added as permanent members of the team. They report, as team members, to the unit manager. This organization decreases the amount of time required for scheduling, coordinating, and waiting for these therapists to provide treatments, and it enhances the skills of all the team members. When diagnostic services such as laboratory testing or radiology are heavily utilized, they might be moved to the patient unit. The remaining patients, who are likely to be unscheduled and less predictable, are cared for by the flex team. The flex team has a richer skill mix (more RN and LPN staffing) than the focus team in order to meet the variable patient needs.

In Phase 3, the design phase, the strategy developed in the previous phase was used to begin designing the new patient-focused system. Again, planners were guided by the restructuring principles as well as the cost and service targets. Examples of these targets included (1) an increase from 50 to 90 percent in patient admission to the correct unit, (2) an increase from 25 to 50 percent of caregiver time devoted to direct patient care, (3) a decrease by 50 percent of the average number of caregivers assisting a patient during a four-day hospital stay, and (4) an 80 percent reduction in redundancies.

The task forces generated ideas, discussed findings, and developed recommendations, action plans, and timetables. Each unit task force decided how to group its patients, then analyzed the extent of utilization of other services based on the patient population's needs. After conducting a cost/benefit analysis, the task force made decisions on moving these services to the patient unit, and the design of the care team began. The cost targets required leveraging the skill mix — that is, using professional staff for professional work and using less-skilled persons for work that did not require professional training — as well as increasing the flexibility of all the team members through multiskilling. Throughout the process, task-force members continually discussed findings with and obtained feedback from the unit staff before developing plans.

Do-it groups (DIGs), comprised of both task-force members and unit or other service staff, performed short-term assignments from the task forces. For example, a DIG might be assigned to explore unit design, to do a study of the amount of laboratory work performed on a unit daily, or to create new position descriptions.

Task forces reported their recommendations to the steering committee for approval. If cost and service targets were not met, the task force was instructed to return to the drawing board and find alternative solutions. Also, the steering committee helped resolve any impasses that task-force members were unable to resolve on their own. Once their plans were accepted, the task forces were dissolved.

At St. Charles the objectives for Phase 4, the implementation phase, were to ensure implementation of the restructuring plans, to provide monitoring systems to manage operations, to continue to process improvement ideas, and to develop management systems and processes to institutionalize continuous improvement.

A tremendous amount of work remains to be done at St. Charles in the implementation phase: new multiskilled workers need to be trained; physical and structural changes need to be made; new equipment needs to be purchased; hiring issues need to be resolved; and interviews need to be conducted to fill new positions. Other issues that need to be resolved include devising new mechanisms for charging for unit-based ancillaries and other budgetary concerns as well as methods to continually evaluate and improve on the new model.

Implementing Care Teams. St. Charles utilized an organizational-development consultant, IMPAQ, to help with implementation of the patient-focused-care teams. They found that developing multidisciplinary teams requires a great deal of energy, knowledge, and skill. Key concerns were to provide safety, support, and structure for the staff. Mark Samuel, president of IMPAQ, outlined a structured approach for this process.

Stage 1: Managers must have a shared vision, be well-coordinated, and feel supported by their own team if they are to provide clear guidance and support for their departments. The management team worked on building commitment and on developing an overall strategy for how the process would work and what individuals would be doing. Specific details of operations were worked out, such as communication and information-flow agreements and strategies for individual and group meetings. In addition, concerns were identified and interaction agreements were developed for a management support system.

Stage 2: Because the department teams were being reorganized, they felt the most insecure. They had to create a support system for themselves in order to avoid isolation or fighting among themselves. During this stage concerns were identified and interaction agreements were made regarding how members would support each other. In addition, members clarified their relationship with their leader and determined how they could support other departments. Also, values and standards were identified, and information-flow processes were developed.

Stages 3 and 4 were implemented during the transition period. During this time people needed to maintain their identity while gaining an understanding of how they would function and operate with their new peers.

Stage 3: People who would be coming onto the new patient-focused team and their new and old managers identified issues of concern and described roles and responsibilities in detail. Also, needs for information and support from outside the group and ways the group could offer support to others were identified. During this stage the group was encouraged to identify critical success factors — that is, values they wanted to maintain as they went into the new team. For example, occupational and physical therapists identified their need to attend OT and PT department meetings in order to stay current in their profession.

Stage 4: During this stage, teams set the stage for building trust among themselves. At team-building retreats, members shared their vision of their new roles, including their daily functions and the percentage of time spent in each area. Knowledge and skill gaps were identified as foundations for education and support plans. As a result, St. Charles added education on delegation, legal issues, time management, supervision, coordination, and adult education. They also developed a follow-up system to review agreements and continue problem solving.

Stage 5: This stage occurred three to six months after Stage 4 began. With trust established and operations more stable than in the beginning, the team could support a common purpose and identity. During this stage the team reviewed and celebrated its successes and developed the team vision, values, and standards. Also, the team assessed its relationships and revised its interaction agreements; at the same time it developed improvement goals and projects with action plans. In addition, it devised a plan for assisting other departments through the transition. Finally, CQI systems were introduced.

Stage 6: This stage was critical for establishing a learning environment, which assists the team in improving results and responding to the ongoing process. This stage includes continual assessing of results, celebrating success, and developing external assessments. Based on these findings new projects and action plans are developed as appropriate.

In addition, processes need to be developed to monitor operations and help the patient-centered teams stay on course. Both quality and service targets need to be continually tracked and used as feedback to improve the system. Monitoring tools need to be identified and developed as well as a system for assuring ongoing monitoring and feedback.

The process outlined above combines a top-down with a bottom-up approach. At least 300 of the 1,100 employees of the St. Charles staff were involved in the restructuring process. The philosophy was to involve employees and have them do as much as possible.

Bishop Clarkson Memorial

At the 1991 Patient-Focused Healthcare Delivery Symposium hosted by the Healthcare Forum, Kevin Moffitt, administrative manager of neurosensory services at Bishop Clarkson Memorial in Omaha, reported that his hospital employed more of a top-down approach than St. Charles. Clarkson utilized consultants and a few hospital personnel working under administrative direction. This group served as the decision-making body. It interacted with a few committees whose job was to react to decisions already made. In designing a second unit Clarkson utilized more of a team approach. In their experience, the team approach takes longer because team members find it difficult to divorce themselves from their old paradigm.

Lee Memorial

Nathan, Hudson, Strazis, and Gomberg (1991) describe the QUEST (Quality, Unity, Education, Service, and Technology) process at the 628-bed Lee Memorial Medical Center in Fort Myers, Florida, as having five phases. In Phase 1, project start-up and planning, a team of twelve consultants and hospital staff began their work by studying the hospital's mission and customers' perceptions and expectations. During this phase the team focused on developing a hospitalwide definition of values that would be used to guide the process.

In Phase 2, the "as is" assessment phase, the team looked at operations by studying the process flows of ten groups of ten to fifteen patients each. They examined everything that affected the patients, from admission to discharge. Using this information, they analyzed how different departments and processes affected patient flow, and they performed a value-added and non-value-added analysis.

Phase 3, development of the "to be" model, was a bottom-up process. Information from the "as is" studies was reviewed and analyzed. Like other hospitals, Lee Memorial found that resources and demand were not synchronized, that many care-giver activities did not add value, and that the flow through the hospital system was less than optimal. Based on the data gathered, it established bench marks for evaluating the process. Using a strong case mix and a cost accounting system, it sorted patients based on resource consumption. Through this process, it was able to determine which test procedures, equipment, and skill levels were needed in the care centers. The resulting "to be" model resembles the model developed at Lakeland.

Phase 4, the implementation phase, was similar to the process other hospitals used.

Phase 5, the "go forward" phase, is devoted to planning

how to establish the "to be" model hospitalwide. This phase involves proactively managing the regulatory issues, investing in training, budgeting for information systems and technology, and challenging the status quo.

The structure for change at Lee Memorial has several components. A steering committee, consisting of physician leaders, administrative staff, and project team members, provides guidance and direction. A change-management committee, consisting of key department directors who act as "change champions," provides assistance in communicating project goals. And departmental advisory teams (consisting of 175 employees) inform the process through their expertise. Lee Memorial believes in staff participation and builds on these formal committees by conducting monthly meetings of employee focus groups to discuss concerns and share ideas and concepts. Other creative processes include a game demonstrating the advantages of locating products and services around the customer and a performance by care coordinators of a vignette about streamlining processes.

According to John Skalko, assistant vice-president for operations improvement, model development began in July 1990 with the orthopedics service because it was a strategic area, had good physician support, and was a fairly straightforward specialty from a care standpoint. The model of the orthopedic unit evolved through the process described above; it includes the following components: admissions/preadmissions testing, pharmacy, laboratory, radiology, multiskilling (phlebotomy, simple respiratory therapy, EKGs), and work simplification (charting-by-exception, flat charging, and implementing the PYXIS system for dispensing narcotics and intravenous-therapy supplies).

After analysis of the various components of the orthopedics model, Lee Memorial identified those that provide the greatest opportunities for operations improvement from a cost/benefit and quality standpoint. According to Skalko, these components are primarily in the work-simplification and multiskilling areas, although the hospital may, after additional analysis, further decentralize ancillary service, such as the pharmacy, laboratories, and radiology.

The three-to-four-year plan includes development of nine

centers: orthopedics, rehabilitation, cardiology, maternal/child, trauma/neurology, medical, surgical, same-day surgery, and outpatient emergency. The goals for these centers are to meet patients' and physicians' expectations for quality service, to create a healthy team environment, and to reduce the cost of providing care.

Managing the Emotional
Side of the Change Process

People involved in a change process can be compared to people going through the process of grieving; they experience the same stages of denial, followed by resistance and acceptance; those going through change experience two additional stages: exploration and commitment (Scott and Jaffe, 1991). These stages of change are as necessary as they are predictable: they signify a transition from the old to the new. The danger lies in ignoring or denying these phases because they are painful; however, not acknowledging and not preparing for these changes results in even more pain and the danger that the process may fail or that talented people may leave. The first stage, denying that the change will occur, is an attempt to ignore the fact that the present way of operating is over. The typical response to this stage is to withdraw and to do the minimum to get by. The best response to this stage is compassionate listening and clear information.

During the next stage, resistance, individuals are concerned with perceived loss—loss of the old ways of operating, loss of control, loss of the familiar. People may be angry, may be depressed, and often feeling unfairly treated. This phase is especially pronounced in hospitals because of the attachment professional caregivers have to their procedures and rituals as well as their bonding with peers. They believe that traditional practices are necessary for successful patient care. They are suspicious of any new methods or models that may jeopardize the success of the past. First-line supervisors, nursing department heads, and other department heads resist change as much as or more than others. They need to be allowed to experience these feelings while still being facilitated through the change. As one nurse complained despite reassurance about the security of her job, "I need to be allowed to be angry about this now; I don't want you to explain away my fears." When the expression of concerns and emotions is discouraged, people often respond with increased resistance, or they suppress these natural feelings, which often diminishes the energy needed to move forward.

Eventually, when the resistance stage is handled effectively, the person moves into acceptance and a shift toward a positive view. This acceptance marks the transition to the next phase, exploration, which is characterized by discovery and learning. Individuals are now ready to welcome the new and begin to work with the change rather than against it. The job of the leaders is to encourage the enthusiasm and feeling of ownership that are beginning to grow. Leaders must acknowledge the ideas and suggestions that are emerging or run the risk of the reemergence of fear and resistance. The goal in this phase is to encourage ownership so that each employee feels a responsibility for changing the culture, challenging the existing structure and policies of the hospital, and developing solutions to recurring problems.

The final stage of the change process is commitment: a time for adopting the new patterns and new ways and celebrating success. At this stage, individuals are ready to embrace change and commit themselves to the organization. When they have been supported and facilitated through the change, they can accept it as inevitable and can accept the new organizational life.

Research on the characteristics of individuals who cope well with change indicates that they feel in control and tend to focus on what they can change rather than being anxious about what they cannot control. These individuals are committed to the goals of the organization, they see change as a challenge rather than a threat, and they feel connected to other people as sources of support. Organizations undergoing change must foster these attitudes in people. Change cannot be limited to a few departments. The entire culture must become dedicated to innovation and continuous improvement. To restructure patient-care delivery and not the administrative level will not be tolerated without scorn from employees. All three levels — individual, team, organization — must be involved in change. If not, the process may be stalled or fail.

Here are some guidelines for managing the human side of the change process:

1. Acknowledge feelings and concerns and encourage people to express them. This acknowledgement does not necessarily mean you agree but that you affirm others' right to have feelings.

2. Listen. Peoples' statements provide valuable information about what they want. Often, these statements contain information that can be used to improve the plan.

3. At the same time, be clear about how the information and ideas will be used. For example, is the leader consulting with the group to obtain information for a decision the leader will make, or is the decision already made and the group is being asked for ideas on how to implement it? It is important that the group be clear about their role in the change process from the start.

4. Validate feelings. Use statements like "I hear your anger" and "I understand this is hard."

5. Explore the concerns behind the feelings.

6. Keep agreements. Doing so shows concern and assures that agreements will not be forgotten.

7. Provide clear information about what is happening.

8. Encourage involvement and participation.

9. Teach the skills that employees need to cope in the new environment. For example, teach employees how to conduct meetings, solve problems, manage conflict, make decisions, and be accountable.

10. Form groups and task forces that are cross-functional, consisting of people from different professions and departments.

11. Do not change everything at once, and take time for renewal and caring for self.

Problems and Lessons Learned

Transforming the organization's human relationships is the key to patient-focused restructuring. Hospitals that have undertaken restructuring have learned the importance of these components of the process: guiding individuals through the change process, exceptional and nearly constant communication, new ways of addressing the blurring and blending of professional and non-professional roles, the standardization of the training for multi-skilled workers, celebrations of success, and the institutionalization of ongoing change. Issues that need to be resolved include whether to involve staff in work redesign and whether the product is worth the pain.

The need for strong leadership is apparent throughout the process. Because this change is such a paradigm shift, all departments need inspiring leadership so that individuals will feel supported enough to give up the security of the past and move into the new paradigm. Any leadership weaknesses or failure to share a common vision quickly leads to disillusionment with the process. If there is lack of agreement on the necessity for change or if management is not convinced of the advantages of change, the process will falter.

A plan for dealing with fears and concerns about change is needed so that people feel comfortable expressing their feelings while the process keeps moving forward. At one hospital a manager spoke up during a meeting of department heads and questioned the process. Her concerns were listened to and addressed in a nonjudgmental way. The reasons for implementing the process were explained and the manager was asked for her commitment to seeing the process through. The manager confided that she had doubted the organization's commitment, but now she was "on board." She further explained, "Yes, I was passing on information, but I didn't have much enthusiasm. I think my staff knew that, and they haven't really bought in yet either." This episode demonstrates the importance not only of allowing concerns to be expressed but also of convincing managers of the need for change so that they can support their staff and gain their staff's support.

During the 1991 Patient-Focused Healthcare Delivery Forum nearly every administrator presenting highlighted the need for nearly continuous communication (*The Healthcare Forum,* 1991). Communication needs to be both factual and inspirational. Communication of data, facts, and targets helps ground the process and gives it a common focus. For example, at St. Charles some nurses found it difficult to think of delegating some of their tasks to less-skilled workers. It was helpful to discuss the research review of the American Nurses Association (1992), which found that 50 percent of nurses' jobs can be delegated to less-skilled workers. It is equally important to communicate clearly when decisions are made and to explain the underlying data supporting them. At St. Charles each new task force had to be provided with relevant data and the opportunity to analyze them on its own. It was easy to forget after the first task force created its design that each succeeding task force needed the same preparation and opportunity to form its own conclusions as well as to learn the skills and data-analysis techniques. At times the failure to provide this opportunity led to resistance and anxiety.

Communication needs also to deal with emotional issues, such as acknowledging and supporting staff in the grief, anxiety, and fear engendered by the change process. St. Charles provided management "roamers" for this purpose. The roamers were instructed in listening skills and were careful not to be too quick to reassure in the face of the unknown. Sometimes, they acted simply as sounding boards, someone to be angry at. They helped open up the communication process and demonstrated to many that the organization cared for them. They were particularly appreciated on the night shift. Often nurses would say, "It's so helpful to have someone just listen to me."

Administrators must also be willing to be vulnerable themselves. Often staff members feel they are the only ones with fears and concerns about change; it is important to demonstrate that administrators also have their concerns. Lussier, the CEO at St. Charles, demonstrated the power of this vulnerability when he addressed an angry group during one of the staff updates. "I have fear related to this change too. I have been an administrator for eighteen years. I had my work down pat. Now, everyone is changing the rules on me. I feel like I have to start all over. I have a vision for what can be and I am committed to guiding us through these turbulent times. Yet, if this doesn't work out who do you think will lose their job?" The staff immediately softened and began asking questions for clarification instead of offering angry accusations.

Also, when people are under stress, they need specific, detailed information, and they need more structure and guidance than they do when they are not under stress. Speaking in generalities and offering global visions only increase the level of stress. One of the greatest challenges is supplying detailed information about what specific employees and departments will be doing in the new system.

One of the most disturbing issues for people is the blurring of professional and nonprofessional identities. As ancillary staff are asked to leave their departments to join patient-focused-care teams, there is a great deal of concern about how they will maintain their professional identity and comradery. Kreitner (1992) explains how Reading Rehab in Pennsylvania is responding to this need: "We have been developing 'virtual' organizations—for each of the clinical specialties (PT, OT, Speech, etc.). The virtual organizations focus on matters other than service delivery, such as professional development and facilitating mentoring relationships." Other hospitals have created regular meeting times for these decentralized professionals so that they can maintain their professional networking.

Hand in hand with the blurring of professional identities is the issue of licensing and certification. It is important for hospitals to work with professional licensing agencies, but they need to be careful not to give away the power and opportunity to create improved delivery systems. Health care cannot afford niches of specialization. If professionals choose to continue to protect their turf and resist change, they may find they are no longer affordable. For example, St. Charles Medical Center and other hospitals throughout Oregon are working with their State Board of Nursing to expand the training and functions of certified nursing assistants.

Nurses, who have essentially performed all functions related to patient care, also struggle with the concept of releasing some of their tasks to multiskilled workers. This concern has two components. First, they are accustomed to integrating nursing process and the performance of care tasks. It takes time and careful work to help them see the value of releasing these tasks to free up time for nursing process and teaching. Second, they may lack the skills and knowledge to be comfortable in delegating and assigning care to other team members. This component can be addressed through education and support.

Professions must take a proactive rather than a reactive stance in guiding their members through these turbulent times. Because nearly every profession is experiencing shortages, it makes good sense to review what can be done by less-skilled persons. The days of specialization and narrowly defined roles are over. The American Organization of Nurse Executives models the kind of leadership needed in its support for the use of unlicensed assistive personnel: "Regulations mandate that R.N.s are responsible and accountable for the nature and quality of nursing care delivery to patients. But, unlicensed assistive personnel can give nurses extra pairs of hands, enabling nurses to use cognitive skills to assess the patient and plan with other care providers to improve patient outcomes" (Miller, 1992).

A big concern for all involved in patient-focused restructuring is the need for standardization of training for multiskilled workers. This is a concern because each hospital is designing the multiskilled worker's role based on its own needs. Because most hospitals have created their own training programs, the education provided to multiskilled workers is as varied as the organizations that employ them. This type of in-house training is expensive and makes it difficult for multiskilled workers to find employment in other settings if they need to. The lack of support from nursing licensing boards and other professional organizations has made it difficult for colleges and universities to add on programs to meet this need. St. Charles has addressed this concern in the short term by working with the local community college. This college provides training for certified nursing assistants, and the hospital will add its own on-site training

in phlebotomy and other skills. Vanderbilt University Medical
Center in Nashville is encouraging its nursing school to develop
a program specifically for multiskilled workers.

In many ways the process of restructuring is a greatly
speeded-up CQI process. It is important to continue systems
and processes that enhance the organization's comfort with ongoing change. In the future it will be crucial to find ways to
institutionalize the multidisciplinary, multilevel groups used to
create the restructuring process. These groups can continue the
work of analysis, idea processing, hypothesis formation and testing, as well as planning and implementation.

Finally, it is just as important to celebrate accomplishments as it is to do the work. Sometimes we can get so busy
that we forget this important part of the process. The celebration of accomplishments and recognition of everyone's hard work
provide a valuable source of energy to fuel the process. These
celebrations can be integrated into meetings or done separately
at appreciation dinners or staff retreats.

Although the importance of these components of the change
process is obvious, other issues are not so clearly resolved. Staff
involvement in work redesign is controversial. Even though staff
involvement helps ensure that staff members will accept change,
there is no guarantee that staff will believe they are creating the
change. At St. Charles the natural resistance to the process led
staff to suspect that everything was already decided and they
simply were not being told. Unfortunately, late in the process
St. Charles learned the importance of being clear about who
is making the final decision when initiating a task force. For
example, in some cases task force members thought they were
making the final decisions when in reality they were acting in
a consultative position to the steering committee, which made
the final decision. This lack of clarity caused unnecessary frustration for the staff and undermined their trust that their ideas
and input were valued. Another drawback was that because the
staff was creating the change, there were no answers in advance
of what the change would be. Often frustration resulted when
questions regarding what the new teams would look like or what
shift hours would be or how many people would be displaced
could be answered only in generalities.

McDonagh, president at St. Joseph's, reports a similar experience. "We opted in the beginning to let our staff design much of this patient centered model. That caused much consternation for the type of people that have trouble with ambiguity. . . . In other words, while ideas brewed and evolved some folks wanted it all written down, concrete and done! Not possible. Even though this ambiguity caused anxiety, I still think it is more valuable to have staff design the program because they know best" (1991, message 639). Also, it takes additional time for staff involvement, and stress increases when staff from different work areas need to leave assignments to serve on task forces. Yet, all in all, we believe the benefits outweigh the burdens of staff involvement.

Are the results of the process worth the pain? Even though the results of patient-focused restructuring have not been in effect long enough for us to be certain of their benefits, most hospitals answer this question in the affirmative. Although many of these hospitals are citing improvements in cost and service as noted in Chapter Two, they warn that this is a long-term process and that returns on investments may not be realized for several years. Yet, benefits are achievable early on. Rick Martin, vice president of operations for St. Charles Medical Center, was pleased to report to the community that, as a result of hospitalwide restructuring efforts, they were able to reduce their rate increase by almost one-half (from 9 percent for January 1992 to 4.5 percent for January 1993). There are many other benefits of the restructuring process. For example, it sets the stage for a natural entry into CQI. The process itself forces positive changes such as ongoing communication at all levels of the organization, the use of data to make decisions, the collection and meaningful presentation of data, and the recognition of empowered, cross-functional teams. Equally important are the transference of management engineering language and principles to hospitals and the recognition of the value of active staff participation in decision making.

Nevertheless, the fast pace of the restructuring process can be exhausting. In the beginning I (Nancy Moore) felt we at St. Charles were going too fast. Bellaire, our consultant, replied to my request to slow the process down. "This kind of major organizational change effort will not succeed if approached on an incremental basis. You have to build enough momentum to overcome resistance and the historical barriers protecting the old system." I soon learned the wisdom of his words. Once we started the process, it became clear that it was important to complete it as soon as possible so staff would know what to expect and be relieved of some of their anxiety. It is important to get models operating as quickly as possible to give staff tangible visions to project themselves into. Also, clearly, in the fast-changing world of today it is important to institutionalize comfort with ongoing change. McDonagh informs us, "While I recognize the need to be sensitive to the effects of change on people, I feel we cannot slow down! We will fall in turbulent waters for sure. . . . I always recommend to folks that rather than slow down the change or halt the momentum of the transformation process, . . . planned rest periods and escapes should be built into the process. Everyone involved in change needs to escape for a while to reenergize and then come back onto the flow to boost everyone else up" (1991, message 350).

The following are some of the recommendations other hospitals have made for those beginning restructuring (as cited by Sasenick, 1992b). From Fairview Hospital and Healthcare System (total of 1,480 beds at four sites, Minneapolis):

1. Start with a compelling strategy or relate restructuring to a problem. Link restructuring to the challenges the organization faces.
2. Work to obtain buy-in of all concerned.
3. Doug Robinson, senior vice president, advises, "An attitude that is helpful is that there are no sacred cows, and that no stones will be left unturned. . . . This message of fairness and the emphasis [on] working as a team [are] important."
4. Institutionalize the change by revising and deleting policies and job descriptions.

From John C. Lincoln Hospital (236 beds, Phoenix):

1. Work to create trust and a willingness to experiment.
2. Be willing to invest in training in both interpersonal and work skills. Consider mentoring and coaching programs to assist staff in their new roles.
3. Support employees in voicing their opinions; at the same time hold them accountable for creating solutions to the problems they identify.
4. Carry through with the process by creating new management models and compensation strategies, such as skill-based pay structures and incentives such as gain sharing.

From Lee Memorial Medical Center (627 beds, Fort Myers, Florida):

1. Be sure you have the financial stability to undertake a project of this magnitude.
2. Determine whether you have these cultural characteristics: "strong and visionary leadership; a cohesive, innovative management team; . . . progressive nursing leadership and organization; and good medical-staff relations."
3. Be proactive in addressing regulatory and union issues.
4. "Drive change from the top and build the model from the bottom up."
5. Be willing to invest in training.
6. Communicate the vision clearly and constantly. Sell the project on a continuous basis.

Putting Patients First

Patient-focused restructuring is a courageous and visionary response to the crisis of cost and of purpose facing health care. It is a fundamental and philosophical change in the very fabric and substance of the hospital. We can envision new organizational charts, as Kaiser has foretold, that are circular and have the patient at the center. There will be no need for boxes and lines as everyone will be united in the common purpose of caring for the patient.

In this chapter we have presented a map for implementing patient-focused care. In closing, we quote Lathrop (1991, p. 20): "Few will challenge the goals of the patient-focused hospital. Many will question the means—telling us 'you can't get there from here.' The simple imperative is: We must get there, and here is the only place we can start. As long as we keep patients and common sense foremost in our minds, we will succeed." In the next chapter we will further explore patient-focused care as we turn to the health care team.

Chapter 5

Health Care Teams in the Patient-Focused Hospital

> Profound and powerful forces are shaking and remaking our
> world, and the urgent question of our time is whether we can
> make change our friend and not our enemy.
>
> William Jefferson Clinton,
> Presidential Inaugural Address, 1993

Patient-focused care has profound implications for the
health care team. Even though most health care providers chose
their work because they were sincerely committed to caring for
people, they often find that the system they are in focuses on
itself instead of on the patient. We begin this chapter by looking at the problems generated by the present system of care delivery, as we focus on the traditional system's effects on its care
providers: nurses, physicians, ancillary staff, support staff, and
care teams. Then we identify two major concerns that any new
approach must address: the decreasing supply of professionals
and the need to improve quality while lowering costs. Next we
present new approaches to care delivery and offer examples of
innovative efforts now under way, such as nursing case management and a variety of nurse-extender models. Finally, we
explore the implications of patient-centered care for management, as we present characteristics of patient-centered management and offer examples of its implementation.

Hospitals are not alone. Old forms are breaking up in
nearly every sector of society. Restructuring is the word for the
time. State governments are restructuring, education systems
are restructuring, and business organizations of all kinds are

restructuring. Professions, too, are called to restate their purposes to conform with new, restructured systems. The traditional hospital developed at a time of cost-based reimbursement and emphasis on the special interests of professions. As new technologies and specialists entered the system, new professions and departments were created. Each profession viewed the patient through its own lens, from its own point of view. The focus and knowledge base of each specialty were the bases for dividing the patient into a multitude of body systems and functions. For example, some hospitals have teams whose sole responsibility is the administration of intravenous fluids. As health care changed, professionals assumed additional responsibilities, without evaluating their work to see whether all tasks were still relevant. As a result, hospitals evolved into systems so complex that none of their constituents are being well served today.

Effect of the Traditional System on Health Care Providers

Nurses leave work stressed and frustrated because they have too little time to meet patient needs.

Ancillary staff, such as pharmacists, physical therapists, and respiratory therapists, resent having to compete with nurses and other professionals for patient-care time.

Support services, such as housekeeping and central supply, feel estranged and demeaned by a system that excludes them from the patient-care team.

Physicians report frustration with bureaucratic responses to their needs and inconsistency in their patients' care.

And patients and families, in this system, are more an afterthought than the center of care.

All of this despite the fact that caring for patients, being part of the vibrant and sacred nature of their healing, is the reason most health care providers entered their professions in the first place.

Nurses

Nurses have been telling us for years that the system is not working, that they spend more time nursing the system than they do nursing patients. Consistently, research (Weber, 1991; Henderson and Williams, 1991a; and Peter Drucker as cited by Flower, 1991) has shown that only 21 percent to 29 percent of what nurses do has anything to do with nursing. Few nurses enter their profession to be clerks. Yet, a full 29 to 50 percent of their time is spent on paperwork (Pronsati, 1992; Lathrop, 1991). The paperwork burden and the increasing demands of technology have served to distance nurses from the core of patient care. Nursing, by definition, provides holistic care through touching, listening, consoling, and teaching, as well as treating — all elements integral to healing. Nurses are well aware that patients define quality by how well their psychosocial needs are met and how promptly they are responded to. Yet nurses often have too many technical and bureaucratic tasks to do to meet patient needs.

Unfortunately, during the 1980s hospitals cut costs by decreasing support staff, only to add to the burden and fragmentation of nurses' work. Added responsibilities increased both the demand for professional nurses and the stress of their work environment. Furthermore, they contributed to excessive work loads, frequent overtime, decreased levels of job satisfaction, and increased turnover rates (O'Malley and Llorente, 1990).

An added source of nurses' frustration is what O'Malley and Llorente (1990) call nursing-role conflict. The major source of this conflict is the system's lack of support for the professional practice of nursing. This lack of support is reflected in the failure of the system to allow nurses time for patient care, to support nurses technologically, and to enforce professional codes of conduct. Cox's (1991) study of verbal abuse suggested that nurses are subjected to condescension, temper tantrums, scapegoating, and public humiliation. The major source of verbal abuse continues to be physicians. Verbal abuse of nurses leads to feelings of powerlessness and incompetence, and decreased self-worth. Lack of respect and verbal abuse by physicians and supervisors are listed as the third most common reason nurses leave their profession (Sigardson, 1982). Nurses have struggled for years in a system that has failed to recognize their value.

But the sword cuts both ways. Nurses, though eager to be recognized as professionals, have not articulated what nursing is. This lack of definition, combined with their failure to speak in one clear voice, has left nurses subject to the domination of other, more powerful professions. Friedman (1991) speaks to the uncertainty of nursing's future. "Nursing continues to struggle with the same issues that have plagued it for 100 years; what nursing is, who should practice it, [with] what preparation, and in what setting." She goes on: "But, because nursing — whatever it is — is so essential to health care, its problems can easily become the problems of health care as a whole" (p. 13).

The link between nursing and health care is described succinctly by Leininger (1986, p. 3): "Nursing is caring; caring is the heart of nursing; and care can be a powerful means for healing and promoting healthy life ways." The health care system has only recently opened its eyes to the distinction between caring and curing and acknowledged that health care is more than medical care. In the American health care system, nurses frequently do the caring and the curing. Nurses outnumber physicians by three to one. In the hospital setting, nurses spend twenty-four hours a day caring for patients, whereas patients spend less than an hour with their physicians during a typical five-day hospital stay (Gordon, 1993, p. 79). In the community setting, nurse practitioners have quietly cared for patients since the 1960s. In an evaluation of their care, the Congressional Budget Office summarized dozens of studies to conclude: "Nurse practitioners have performed as well as physicians with respect to patient outcomes, proper diagnosis, management of specialized medical conditions, and frequency of patient satisfaction" (cited in Gordon, 1993, p. 81). Furthermore, the Office of Technology Assessment found that patients were even more satisfied with nurse practitioners than with physicians. The researchers attributed this satisfaction to nurse practitioners' advanced communication, counseling, and interviewing skills (Gordon, 1993).

Nevertheless, the breadth and depth of nursing have left it vulnerable to the criticism that it is diffuse and unfocused. The need for a powerful nursing voice has never been greater. Walter Cronkite (as cited by Gordon, 1993, p. 82) described the situation quite clearly during a recent PBS special: "Our health care system is neither healthy nor caring, it is not even a system. Recognition of nurses' expertise and importance is critical to changing that."

Another factor contributing to the nonrecognition of nursing as a profession is that nurses can have different levels of educational preparation. Nursing degrees include an associate degree, a bachelor of science, a master's, a nurse practitioner degree, and a doctorate. All these levels of education share a common focus on nursing process, theory, and caring, yet nurses at each level offer a unique perspective based on their education, expertise, and degree of independence of practice. For example, nurse practitioners are required to have a master's degree and additional training that allows them to diagnose, treat, and prescribe for medical conditions while under the supervision of a physician, whereas the associate-degree nurse utilizes the nursing process and follows orders prescribed by the physician.

Sadly, nursing's greatest strength is also its weakness. Nursing's dedication to caring and patient-focused care has been interpreted as weakness or lack of professionalism by some. Because nurses have remained, by and large, at the bedside and resisted putting their energies into political action and articulation of their profession's stature, nursing is at risk of looking weak and ill defined. Clearly, with estimates that increased reliance on nonphysician practitioners would save U.S. consumers about $90 billion each year in medical costs (Gordon, 1993), nurses need to be far less humble and more assertive in promoting their profession. Gordon (1993, p. 82) tells us, "They [nurses] also need advocates and allies — among patients, families, politicians, businesspeople, and journalists — who understand that high-quality health care is dependent not only on technology, fancy surgery, and the promise of cure, but also on the efforts of hundreds of women and men who provide the care without which the cure would be impossible."

Ancillary Staff

Strasen (1991) reports that personnel in ancillary departments such as physical therapy, respiratory therapy, occupational therapy, social services, and pharmacy spend 40 percent of their time "going to" or "waiting to" provide services to patients. Once they connect with patients, they are limited to performing a specific task. This fragmented approach prevents them from seeing how their treatment affects patients' overall outcomes.

Ancillary staff long for a relationship with other team members that promotes continuity of care. After the implementation of patient-focused care at Lee Memorial Hospital in Fort Myers, Florida, Patrick Arthur, physical therapy supervisor, reported, "Previously, therapists would leave the [physical therapy] department and go to the orthopedic floor to treat patients there. Locating the appropriate chart often was time-consuming, and because the notes were lengthy and somewhat complicated, the [physical therapists] also spent a significant amount of time bringing themselves up to date on each patient's status" (quoted in Pronsati, 1992, pp. 5-6). Arthur also reported that therapists frequently left frustrated after arriving to perform a treatment and finding the patient involved in another procedure, gone from the room, or in need of pain medication. With a patient-focused approach, Arthur says, "You have assurance the patient will be in the room and ready for your visit because the primary care team will know to expect you. . . . Interaction is simplified by the fact that you are not dealing with alot of people, but rather the same two teams of three caregivers" (p. 6).

Likewise, pharmacists are frustrated because of the departmental barriers that preclude their providing valuable input for patient care. Isolated in centralized pharmacies and physically out of contact with the patient and the health care team, they miss opportunities to consult with physicians and nurses about pain control, drug interactions, and drug therapies. As a result, the possibility of their making such contributions is often unknown to other professionals. Others cannot appreciate what they have not previously experienced.

When pharmacists are decentralized to patient-care units and available for nurse and physician consultation, not only can patient care improve, but it may also become more cost effective. Pharmacists can provide physicians with information on alternative medications that are equally effective and less costly than their counterparts. As a result of becoming a part of patient-focused-care teams, pharmacists at St. Charles Medical Center report a renewed joy in their work. They enjoy seeing patients and the effect of medicinal treatment, working collaboratively with physicians and nurses, and being appreciated by these team members for their expertise.

Social services personnel are frequently frustrated in trying to do discharge planning in a traditional system. Far too often, they are informed of the need for complex discharge planning the day before or, worse yet, on the day a patient is supposed to go home. The following scene occurs far too often: A social services representative receives a referral for discharge planning. Arriving at the room, she finds a very elderly man lying in bed. During her assessment, she learns he is a widowed farmer who lives alone thirty miles from the city. Unfortunately, he has a wound infection that requires frequent dressing changes and will require intravenous antibiotics for at least one week after discharge. When she asks the nurse why she was not notified earlier, he replies, "I don't know. I just started taking care of him today, and when the doctor mentioned he would go home tomorrow, I realized we were going to need your help. He hasn't changed his own dressing yet, and I don't think anyone has taught him how to give his own antibiotics." Needless to say, such occurrences are frustrating and stressful for social services personnel and obviously can compromise a patient's care.

Another source of job dissatisfaction for social services personnel is the often task-oriented nature of their job. They are trained as professional counselors and often choose their profession because they enjoy counseling and helping people. Yet their traditional role in hospitals is discharge planner, and they find they often spend most of their time making phone calls and locating equipment.

In addition, with the traditional, centralized approach, ancillary personnel miss opportunities to network with, to support, and to learn from each other. Departmental barriers foster an environment where misunderstandings and lack of awareness of each other's work can easily lead to backbiting, complaining, and energy wasted in interdepartmental conflict. Removing artificial barriers and bringing all the key health care players on one team have many benefits for the patient and the team. For example, physical therapists are great resources for caregivers as well as for patients. Hospitals are notorious for work-related injuries. Many of these injuries are back strains caused by poor body mechanics or lack of help in moving weakened patients. With health care's graying workforce, on-site teaching about body mechanics and support in patient care are growing necessities. Also, the counseling and group-facilitation expertise of social services personnel can greatly enrich the holistic approach to patient care and facilitate the growth of the team.

Support Staff

In a centralized system, support personnel feel alienated and unimportant. Yet, consistently, patients report that the quality of the food and the cleanliness of their rooms greatly affect their perceptions of quality of care. Often, patients and family members recall an experience with a housekeeper as significant in their hospital experience. As one family member who had lost a loved one commented, "The person who helped me the most through this was the housekeeper. She would come in every morning, and I could tell by the look in her eyes that she really wanted to help. She would smile and ask how I was doing as she cleaned the room. It meant so much to me to have someone to talk to. And, this sounds funny, but it was so important to have everything clean and tidy. I remember so well, thinking in the elevator, this stainless steel should be sparkling clean. Cleanliness was so important during that time."

Generally, people from support services such as central supply, supply processing and distribution, and food preparation want to be part of patient care. They are eager to be part of a team and to feel they are more than a cog in a machine. Instead, they often feel alienated. Too often most of their interaction with team members is via the phone. These faceless encounters lead to the venting of frustrations that often have nothing to do with support services. For example, nurse Mary calls for a nasogastric tube in a sharp and pressured voice: "I want an NG tube right now. And, I mean now! I'm sick and tired of the service around here!" The receiver of the call breaks into tears or yells back, not knowing the nurse was just screamed at by the physician.

In addition, the separation of these support personnel from their customers makes the true institution of quality and service excellence unlikely or at least difficult. When supply personnel are part of the patient-care team, they anticipate needs and can see how, when, and why supplies are needed. As a result of face-to-face relationships and a total team effort, they report feeling supported by the team, and team members report improvements in their ability to perform their work as a result of innovations contributed by support personnel who now have the total picture.

Physicians

Physicians, the traditional gatekeepers of the system, have warned for some time that hospitals are too bureaucratic and inefficient. The same complaints are heard over and over in medical-staff meetings throughout the country. These complaints include:

- Lack of timely information for decisions. For example, long turnaround times for laboratory and radiology reports may increase the length of hospital stay or compromise patient care.
- Paperwork that is excessive and often meaningless. Physicians as well as other health care providers are frustrated and overburdened by what St. Charles Medical Center calls the "paper blizzard." Hospitals have forms for everything. The duplication of information and sheer complexity of documentation often make it difficult if not impossible to find pertinent information.
- Inefficient systems. Just finding out who is caring for their patients is a time-consuming and sometimes futile task. As one physician commented, "I never see the same nurse twice. And when I ask a nurse for a report on my patient, I often hear, 'I'm sorry, I just started taking care of him today. I don't know if he is improving or not.'"

Another example is the often frustrating attempts of physicians and nurses to contact one another. The endless phone tags and paging are enough to drive anyone to profanity. In a typical scene, nurse Nancy pages Dr. Strong to report that his patient's blood pressure is dropping. Dr. Strong is on his way to his office. There is a ten-minute delay before he can return the call. Meantime, nurse Nancy has left the phone to care for her patient. The phone rings seven times and finally is answered by nurse Jim. He did not page Dr. Strong, and he has no idea who did. Nurse Nancy returns and complains that Dr. Strong did not answer his page. She calls his office. The office nurse replies that he is with a patient and that she will have him return the call. And so it goes—one can only hope that they connect at some point, by which time both nurse Nancy and Dr. Strong will be close to being verbally abusive. And the patient is wondering why no one is attending to his needs.

The implications of this fragmented approach to care go far beyond the discomfort of frustration. Research (Knaus, Draper, Wagner, and Zimmerman, 1986) indicates that patients' lives may depend on collaborative relationships between nurses and physicians as well as continuity of care. Researchers of The George Washington University Medical Center, Washington, D.C., studied treatment and outcome of 5,030 patients in intensive care units at thirteen tertiary care hospitals using diagnosis, indication for treatment, and acute physiology and chronic health evaluation (APACHE) 11 scores. The total APACHE 11 score predicts the chances of each patient's survival. Accuracy of this prediction varied depending on which unit the patient was in. In the units with the "best" outcomes, 55 percent more patients lived than were predicted. In the units with the "worst" outcomes, 58 percent more patients died than were anticipated (p. 410). After careful study of these surprising findings, the researchers concluded that the significant variables between the "best" and "worst" units were collaborative relationships between nurses and physicians based on mutual respect and trust as well as the existence of primary nursing involving nurse autonomy and continuity of care.

Neither health care professionals nor patients can afford

the cost of a fragmented and paternalistic approach to care. In particular, health care professionals must collaborate and respect one another's contributions if they are to survive in a managed-care environment. With this system, everyone gains when each player works collaboratively and efficiently toward the common goal: the health of the patient. Managed-care companies, employers, and patients choose providers with the lowest costs and best outcomes for their clients. Unfortunately for physicians, managed care means they are no longer the gatekeepers to the system.

Even without the influence of managed care, the physician's role is changing. Goldsmith and Miller (1990) comment on the complexity of patient care today: "The real doctor for a chronically ill elderly patient today is not . . . the physician . . . but the multidisciplinary team . . . whom that physician relies on for advice and management help" (p. 28). Most care of patients with chronic illnesses is being organized around the team model. Such teams provide, for example, diabetic care, cancer care, cardiac care, and rehabilitation.

Care Teams

The success of the team approach with chronically ill patients and the fact that no individual or profession has enough information or expertise to be the sole provider of care make it clear that a team approach is necessary. Yet, structurally, hospitals have precluded true team approaches because of the compartmentalization and specialization of ancillary and support services. Although hospital administrators have touted the need to collaborate and work together, the system's structural barriers, such as department locations and organizational lines of reporting, have subverted all attempts at truly patient-centered care.

The traditional hospital system remains hierarchical. Often, an observer can hear nurses or assistants on a team say, when called to help a patient outside of their specific area, "That's not my patient." The same is true for social services, personnel, physicians, and other ancillary-service personnel, who come and go, feeling little responsibility and accountability for meeting total patient needs.

Today, no one profession can do it all. The best medical staff, nursing department, physical therapy department, and pharmacy do not make the best patient-care environment if they do not blend their efforts into one system.

Concerns

Two major concerns must be addressed in developing new approaches to patient care: a decreasing supply of professionals and the need to improve quality while lowering costs.

Decreasing Supply of Professionals

Hospitals must be sensitive to the dwindling numbers of nurses and other professionals. The U.S. Department of Health and Human Services Secretary's Commission on Nursing (1988) found professional shortages in nearly every sector of health care. At the same time, future availability of these resources is even bleaker because of declining birthrates during the mid-1960s and 1970s. According to Hanrahan (1991), "This puts hospitals on a collision course with the 'age wave' which alone can capsize the system. Hospitals will have to learn to make more intelligent use of their increasingly scarce human resources" (p. 34).

Need to Improve Quality While Lowering Costs

"Who is coordinating all this care? Who is evaluating if the right treatment is being given? Who sees the big picture? As management engineers entered hospitals to assist with restructuring and design, the veil was lifted. Nursing is at the pivotal juncture of quality and cost" (Hanrahan, 1991, p. 37). And the consumer agrees. Inlander and Weiner (1985) advise consumers: "Doctors may make the money, administrators may sign the check, trustees may break ground for new buildings — but nurses run the show. Of everybody you deal with during a hospital stay, nobody is as important, can do more for you (and to you), and can be more a colleague-in-arms than your nurse" (p. 75). Nurses, who are at the heart of the delivery system, must be focused on cost-effective, quality patient care (Tonges, 1992). According to Hanrahan (1991), the challenge for hospitals is to close the growing gap between the need for nurses to assume an empowered role in a redefined system and the pressure for them to remain in the traditional task-oriented role decreed for them by some physicians. The challenge for nursing is to use this opportunity to create a process that focuses on outcome rather than tasks and functional areas such as nursing units and radiology.

New Approaches

Models that blend clinical outcome, economical case management, and a collaborative team approach into operational redesign are urgently needed. Tonges (1992) identifies the desirable features of such a model:

- It leverages skills—that is, it redistributes some aspects of nursing tasks to the lowest appropriate level of caregiver.
- It decentralizes services to the patient-care unit.
- It promotes collaboration among nurses, physicians, and other health professionals. Together care providers develop common pathways of care as case-management tools for streamlining and economizing the delivery of care.

Nursing Case Management

Perhaps the most promising model to meet these challenges is nursing case management, a collaborative model with a set of components for the strategic management of cost and quality. The New England Medical Center Hospitals are recognized as pioneers of nursing case management. They based their model on the following beliefs (Zander, 1988):

1. Nurses have always been responsible for managing patient care; however, they have labored with inadequate tools and systems such as care plans and a shift-centered system.

2. "Quality is definable in terms of a specific clinical process and outcome standards. . . . Quality in healthcare is thus a product, not a service" (p. 28).

3. The true cost of patient care can be understood and revised on a case-type basis using DRGs. The most potentially controllable costs of care lie in the nursing realm because lack of self-care and physical complications (respiratory problems, immobility) can be prevented through careful management.

4. "Nursing makes a major contribution to clinical outcomes through powerful interventions based on diagnostic reasoning and by making the system work for patients and physicians; and nursing allocates much of the hospital's resources" (p. 28).

5. Although nurses and physicians depend on one another, they work in parallel structures. Positive patient outcomes are more likely to be achieved by having formal collaborative-practice groups working with agreed-upon protocols than under the present system. Furthermore, clinicians can benefit from learning management strategies.

Components. This model achieves clinical and financial goals through four components: work design, the use of clinicians as managers, concurrent monitoring in order to provide immediate feedback, and patient and family participation.

Work design includes case-management plans (CMPs) and critical paths. The CMP is a comprehensive protocol for an entire hospital stay. It shows the relationships between a DRG, problems that patients and families are likely to encounter, outcomes, and nursing and physician interventions necessary to achieve these outcomes.

The critical path is an abbreviated form of the CMP. It shows the key incidents and interventions that should occur on a given day to achieve the outcomes within the DRG-allotted length of stay. Critical paths help avoid last-minute oversights, which compromise discharge processes. They also help standardize care and are used as orientation tools for staff, physicians, patients, and families.

Case managers use concurrent monitoring to provide feedback as they note and record deviations from the critical paths, expose the causes, and take appropriate actions. In addition, the records of variances are used for quality-improvement purposes. The data may lead eventually to alterations in the system, practitioners' practice, or patient-treatment protocols. For example, system variations may point to a need for new equipment; practitioners' variations may highlight a need for education; and patient-treatment variations may lead to the development of new care protocols.

The use of clinicians as managers is the key to case management. Through them the work design is converted into outcomes. They are "professionals skilled as both clinicians and managers who are committed to the welfare of both patients and institution" (Zander, 1988, p. 27). They are responsible for developing care for their case load. They revise the CMP based on an assessment of patient needs. Furthermore, they are accountable for effective use of resources, maintaining standards of care, and meeting outcomes within length of stay allotted by the DRG.

To help with the management of individual cases, the New England model uses an ad hoc, episode-based group that consists of nurses and physicians who transcend unit affiliations. This group includes primary nurses from patient-care units, representatives from agencies who provide follow-up care after discharge, and key physicians. Patients and families may also be included. The group discusses individual cases and specific variances from critical paths to identify trends and strategies.

The final component is active patient and family involvement. The process starts on admission as physicians and nurses include patients and their family in discussions of their critical path and variations they can expect. Goals and the methods are negotiated. In addition, resources needed for care are identified in advance of discharge. These practices help clarify for patients and families the activities needed to achieve their desired outcomes. As a result, they are more likely than those who have not been involved to comply with the system's demands, and they are more satisfied with their treatment.

Benefits. Benefits of case management include decreased complications, improved patient and family participation and sense of security, improved physician/nurse relations, decreased lengths of hospital stay, as well as decreased readmissions with their attendant costs.

Zander (1988) reports that after initiating nursing case management for ischemic stroke patients at New England Medical Center Hospitals, clinicians were able to decrease ICU days by 47 percent and the average length of stay by 29 percent. At the same time, they report quality improvement as a result of minimizing the sensory deprivation of patients in ICUs.

The Nursing Network

Another example of nursing case management is the Nursing Network, which reaches into the community. Carondelet St. Mary's Hospital and Health Center in Tucson, Arizona, has implemented the Nursing Network, an integrated system that uses nurses as the primary health care providers. According to Ethridge and Lamb (1989), the Network "produces dramatic reductions in length of stays and cost, while truly 'humanizing' healthcare" (p. 30). Patient care and coordination are the responsibility of a professional nurse case manager (PNCM). The PNCM is at the hub of a full complement of health care components: acute-care inpatient services, extended care/long-term services, hospice service, and ambulatory care services (including traditional physician-directed services and nurse-managed community-based clinics).

Ethridge and Lamb (1989) remark, "The emphasis placed on Professional Nursing Case Management within the Nursing Network signals a commitment to the traditional values and goals of nursing practice, namely, caring for unique individual and family healthcare needs over time. . . . Nurses are available to assist clients to create healing environments, to make choices that lessen disease and to strive for higher levels of health" (p. 35).

The assumptions underlying the Nursing Network (Ethridge and Lamb, 1989, p. 31) are simple: The quality of patient services is directly related to professional accountability, continuity of care, a holistic approach to patient and family needs, and the educational preparation of the nurse providing care.

Distinctive Features. PNCMs carry an active case load of about forty patients, including patients in acute care and in the community. In addition, they may have another forty or fifty patients who are stable and require only monthly telephone calls for evaluation. PNCMs are responsible for patient and family assessment, establishment of nursing diagnoses, and care planning, including delegating tasks to care associates, activating interventions, collaborating with the interdisciplinary team, and evaluating outcomes. They receive referrals from both the community and the hospital and follow their patients and families through the entire process. After discharge, within the home and the community the PNCM assesses needs, provides interventions, teaches about health, consults about health issues, and requests physician and other services for follow-up as needed.

PNCMs can be either unit-based or non-unit-based. Those who are unit-based have specialized expertise, such as in respiratory therapy or oncology, that is needed for managing the care of patients on a particular unit. Non-unit-based PNCMs can manage the care of patients across units and throughout the hospital.

Ethridge and Lamb report excitement about an evolving group-practice model at the Nursing Network. "Members of the group practice collaborate to provide nursing services in an environment that promotes and expects professional accountability" (1989, p. 33). Members of the group, including clinicians, nurse administrators, educators, and researchers, carry an active case load. All members share their different perspectives and expertise within a professional framework to enhance quality and cost outcomes.

Nursing Wellness Centers are community-based clinics where PNCMs provide health information and screening, monitoring, and counseling services for elderly clients. Also, these nurse practitioners coordinate workshops and lectures as well as physician referrals based on their clients' needs. A unique characteristic of this service is its emphasis on the needs of family caregivers as well as of patients. These centers serve the acutely ill in need of posthospital care for recovery; the chronically ill who require ambulatory care or home health services; the terminally ill who require community and hospice support; and high-risk clients who are essentially well but require ambulatory service for disease prevention.

Evaluation. Ethridge and Lamb (1989) report the following results. First, patients and family members have increased confidence in their ability to provide home care, adhere to medication and diet regimes, and adjust to chronic illness.

Second, acuity and lengths of hospital stay are reduced. One study indicated that case-managed patients for total hip replacement had an average length of stay (ALOS) of 8.1 days in comparison with an ALOS of 10.2 days for non-case-managed patients, even though the case-managed patients had a higher acuity. Case-managed patients with chronic illnesses also proved to have a positive financial impact because of decreased hospital stays. "Case-managed patients entered the hospital at a lower acuity level and reduced their length of stay [during] the typical high cost days at the beginning of hospitalization" (p. 33). For respiratory illness the case-managed patients had an ALOS of 6.0 days compared with 9.5 days for the non-case-managed patients.

Cost savings in these cases may be substantial. For example, patients with respiratory disease account for 10 percent of all admissions at Carondelet St. Mary's Hospital and Health Center. Chronic obstructive long disease (DRG 88) is the largest subset of this group. DRG 88 accounted for the largest financial loss to the hospital among Medicare patients. After instituting case management, the tables were turned. As a result of reduced lengths of stay and lesser acuity Carondelet St. Mary's saved $1,552 per case, in addition to cost savings from decreased needs for staffing.

Primary Nursing

Many of these models assume a primary-nursing delivery system. Just as patients have a physician who is primarily responsible for their medical care, with primary nursing they also have a nurse who is primarily responsible for their overall care. The primary nurse assesses patient needs and develops a plan of care; other nurses follow this plan of care when the primary nurse is off duty. At Boston's Beth Israel Hospital patients who are admitted more than once are admitted to the floor where their primary nurse is practicing (Gordon, 1993).

Primary nursing empowered nurses to attain and maintain authority over patient care. It paved the way for nursing to move from a task-based work activity to a knowledge-based profession (Manthey, 1989). Ethridge and Lamb (1989) state that "the continuity and accountability inherent in primary nursing, along with the bonding that takes place between the patient and nurse, are important underpinnings of the case management model" (p. 32).

Clearly, patients benefit from a consistent plan of care and from having decisions made by someone who knows them. Likewise, nurses benefit from consistency and predictability of patient-care assignments. These are among the reasons that Planetree chose a primary-nursing model. In addition, the Planetree philosophy promotes nurse autonomy, which has been shown to enhance job satisfaction (as cited by Martin, Hunt, Hughes-Stone, and Conrad, 1990). And at Planetree the nurses are expected to work collaboratively with other team members, including physicians, nutritionists, and physical therapists.

Managed-Care Teams

Yet, for many hospitals facing financial stresses and shortages of professional nurses, primary nursing is simply not a feasible option. As a result, many hospitals have adapted the New England group model to fit their unique needs and constraints. For example, St. Joseph's Hospital in Asheville, North Carolina, developed managed-care teams because, as in many areas, this region's pool of RNs is limited (Lulavage, 1991). The hospital assigns patients to managed-care teams by case type and uses critical paths to monitor and guide care. In addition, the hospital uses variance reports along with case consultations and team meetings. As a result, the teams systematically monitor, communicate, evaluate, and respond to variances during the course of hospitalization.

Professionally Advanced Care Teams

Similarly, Robert Wood Johnson University Hospital created a Professionally Advanced Care Team (ProACT) (Tonges, 1989a, 1989b, and 1992) as a response to accelerating demands for nursing services, a diminishing pool of professional nurses and other workers, and shrinking financial resources. The Pro-ACT model includes three nursing roles: the clinical-care manager (CCM), the primary nurse, and the licensed practical nurse (LPN). The CCM assesses and coordinates care, ensuring that patient outcomes are achieved in the established time frames. The primary nurse manages the care of a group of patients on a twenty-four-hour basis, participates in direct and indirect care delivery, consults with the CCM regarding patient problems and conditions, assesses patients, establishes priorities and plans, and delegates appropriate tasks to LPNs and nurses' aides. The LPN acts as an associate nurse to the primary nurse and practices under the primary nurse's supervision. The nurses' aides perform tasks that require a lower level of skill. The ProACT model addresses the problem of a diminishing pool of professional nurses by utilizing their skills more wisely. The vacant RN positions and the change in staff mix provided the money for the additional support service personnel and the CCM positions. The hospital anticipates that the recognition of nurses' professional expertise will improve both nurse retention and recruitment.

In addition, the hospital uses a support-services host (SSH). The SSH position integrates the work of several previous positions (housekeeper, dietician, and central-stores clerk) with a number of tasks — answering the phone, calling for supplies, making unoccupied beds, preparing patients for meals, distributing water and linen — previously assumed by a variety of personnel. The hospital also enhanced service by including on the team a unit-based pharmacy technician who assumes responsibility for all medication-related work short of administration.

According to Tonges (1989), the results of the ProACT model include improved satisfaction among nurses as a result of the opportunity to advance to the CCM role, which is more exciting and distinctly different from previous nursing roles; increased ease of integration of ancillary personnel into working groups; and improved satisfaction of support staff as they now feel like part of the team. In addition, staff members' accountability for their work strengthens their self-esteem. Costs with the ProACT model remained the same as previously. Even though there was an overall increase in FTEs, the cost was offset by using a less-rich skill mix.

Nurse-Extender Models

Another natural outgrowth of primary care and limited nursing resources is the nurse-extender model. A nurse extender works as a technical assistant to an experienced RN. In this model, nursing tasks are evaluated and redistributed to less-skilled workers. Unlike the nurses' aide, the nurse extender performs many tasks previously performed by a variety of support staff, including clerical workers, housekeepers, and personnel performing basic clinical functions. According to Hanrahan (1991), nurse extenders have become an essential part of the patient-care process, adding value and satisfaction. The titles and characteristics of nurse extenders are as varied as the organizations that employ them. The following are a few examples.

Practice Partners. Manthey (1989) describes the partner's role as similar to that of a physician's assistant except partners act as an assistant to the nurse. The senior partner (an experienced RN) is responsible for care planning. Also, the senior partner has authority to teach the practice partner decision-making and technical skills within the framework of their state practice act and hospital policies. This arrangement is unique in that compatibility is determined through work-style analysis, and the partners select each other. Partners have included student nurses, certified nurses' aides, and nurses who failed their state board examinations.

According to Manthey (1992), nurses report "comfort, security, and confidence" as a result of "knowing that someone whom they trusted was taking care of patients with them" (p. 18). This model has been effective in the transition of new graduates into acute-care areas. One hospital reported this model decreased orientation time on their neonatal ICU from a year to six months. An added benefit has been solution of the problem of role conflict between RNs and LPNs.

Manthey recommends two guidelines for successful partnerships: (1) At least 75 percent of the total nursing work must fall within the scope of what the partner can do. (2) The work load must be equitably balanced between the two partners.

Patient-Care Assistants. Staff nurses at Alta Bates Herrick Hospital in Berkeley, California, created the position of patient-care assistant in response to their frustration in not being able to meet the comfort and information needs of their patients. Nurses created the job description by listing the tasks they were willing to give up. They retained control of the position by establishing rigid qualifications and an in-house training program. Hanrahan (1991) sites a reduction of $1.3 million in labor costs during 1990 as a result of the new positions.

General Medical Technicians. In order to free up nurses for a higher level of caregiving, HCA West Paces Ferry Hospital in Atlanta created the position of general medical technician (GMT). GMTs are able to perform a variety of tasks under the supervision of an RN. These include such tasks as disconnecting intravenous lines, setting up traction, assisting with physical examinations, and changing dressings. GMTs receive six months of college training to prepare them for the position. As a result, their managers report being able to delegate 44 percent of the activities previously performed by nurses (Hanrahan, 1991).

Unit Assistants. The position of unit assistant was created by Rush Presbyterian St. Luke's Medical Center in Chicago, for the performance of a variety of nonclinical tasks, including materials handling, administration, housekeeping, transportation, and support activities such as changing beds and feeding patients. Cost savings and increased nursing satisfaction were reported by management (Hanrahan, 1991).

Necessity is the mother of invention. Many nurse extender models have evolved out of the need to leverage the skills of costly and scarce professionals and at the same time provide quality patient care. The ones we have described are among the most promising. Now we will turn to the need to create an organizational context that supports empowerment of these care providers.

Implications for Management

Hospitals, like most American organizations, have failed to adapt successfully to today's complex, rapidly changing environment because of an overly bureaucratic approach to management. Joiner (1986) criticizes American management approaches as too focused on short-range quantitative goals, such as short-term cost reduction, quarterly dividends, and market-share growth. At the same time, too little attention has been paid to broader goals, such as quality service, employee involvement, long-range risk taking, and innovation. After reviewing studies of high-performing corporations (Ouchi, 1981; Pascale and Athos, 1981; Deal and Kennedy, 1982; Peters and Waterman, 1982; and Kanter, 1983), Joiner (1986) identifies the new leadership approach as "creating sleeker, more responsive, customer-oriented corporations that stress values like quality, service, and reliability—'operations-driven' organizations that are flexible, decentralized, and have fewer management levels" (p. 41).

Leaders in this organizational climate are people-oriented. They emphasize personal responsibility and recognition, working hard, and having fun. They value teamwork, creativity, initiative, and risk taking. They back up new approaches with lots of training and develop innovative practices, like semiautonomous work groups, and performance-oriented work incentives, like employee stock ownership.

Principles

A Chicago Health Executives Forum task force reported that "success of the patient-focused model is dependent on empowering those involved in direct care" (1991, p. 22). In general, this requirement translates into management's relinquishing some of its authority and sharing responsibility with the actual caregivers. This new organizational environment is characterized by employee participation, commitment, and self-management. This organizational form is best described as a network or circle. It consists of linked groups or teams focused on the center rather than the top (Scott and Jaffe, 1991).

The following characteristics of the traditional hierarchical organization and the new organization of interdependent teams illustrate the shift from one management form to the other.

Traditional Management Style	*Patient-Focused Management Style*
Managers are responsible for outcomes.	Employees are responsible and accountable for outcomes.
Decisions are made by managers.	Decisions are made by the person closest to the patient.
Jobs are clearly defined.	People are flexible and work cooperatively together.
Change is from the top and is generally slow.	Change occurs in response to problems and challenges and occurs quickly.
Communication flows from the top down.	Employees are skilled at giving and receiving feedback.
Communication between departments is minimal.	Interdepartmental communication is prized, and decisions are shared.
The organization has many layers.	The organization has few layers.
Managers tell employees what to do and how to do it.	Managers are facilitators, coaches, connectors, and empowerers of their teams.
Learning is a one-time thing.	Learning is a continuous process. People pay attention to the effects of actions and, as a result of learning, adjust future actions in order to be more effective.

Creating an organizational climate supportive of patient-focused care means creating an environment of responsiveness and commitment to CQI. For patient-focused care to succeed, the structure of the traditional organization must change. The goals are to reduce layers of supervision and to reduce barriers between departments, disciplines, and services that often impede information flow, decision making, prompt response to problems, and collaboration in patient care. Patient-focused structures bring all relevant services to the patient-care unit to form an interdisciplinary team. These teams are challenged to find new ways to work together and to blend their skills while still maintaining their professional identity. In today's health care environment these teams must use CQI, with its emphasis on meeting or exceeding customer expectations, using analysis of data to improve processes, and planning and implementing change on a continuous basis.

The manager's role in patient-focused care is fundamentally different from the traditional manager's role. The traditional unit is managed by an RN who is responsible for about twenty-five to thirty nursing personnel working in collaboration with ancillary departments over which they have no direct authority. On many patient-focused units all ancillary-services personnel, nurses, and other personnel assigned to the unit report directly to the unit manager, who may or may not be an RN. The manager must have knowledge of all ancillary functions and maintain a relationship with central departments. For example, at Bishop Clarkson, the clinical manager has about 100 employees reporting to her (Chicago Health Executives Forum, 1991). With the patient-focused approach, all staff members have increased responsibility for quality and costs. For example, at one hospital, employees spend 10 percent to 40 percent of their time on administrative functions.

Many managers are threatened by the idea of giving up control and sharing power and authority with employees. Some managers need support and education in order to make the transition; others simply do not find the new style compatible with their personalities.

Here are some guidelines for developing participative managers:

1. Develop in managers clear vision, values, standards, and expectations.
2. Provide training programs and discussions for managers, including training in both attitudes and skills. Follow up with mentoring and coaching to help them in the transition.
3. Expect resistance from some managers. Allow time for making the transition; however, replace those who simply cannot or will not change their style. Keep in mind that their values and goals may no longer be compatible with those of the organization. It is in these managers' best interest to find an organization they are compatible with.
4. Institute an evaluation system whereby managers receive feedback from their employees.
5. Create mechanisms to share knowledge, information, accomplishments, new directions, successes, and failures.
6. Value risk taking and learning from mistakes.

The following are overall guidelines for redefining organizational structure and establishing a patient-focused climate:

1. Develop a participative management style that empowers teams.
2. Empower employees to respond directly to customer needs.
3. Educate everyone in CQI, including the philosophy and how to meet and exceed customer expectations, develop quality indicators, study and improve processes, conduct successful meetings, solve problems, make decisions, and manage projects.
4. Flatten the management structure and reduce the number of job classifications. Assign all relevant services to the patient-care unit, bringing them under one manager and into one team focused on the patient.
5. Review and redefine policies and practices regarding career advancement and pay scales. Reward flexibility and teamwork.
6. Develop teamwork, emphasizing accountability and responsibility.

We presented the process for this transformation in Chapter Four.

Models

Now we will review some interesting management models that have many of the characteristics just described.

Shared Governance. The shared-governance model attempts to place accountability at the level of responsibility for practice — in other words, with the staff nurse. Take this example. The evening nurse was upset. Operating rooms had not been stocked, and equipment had not been put away. In the past he would have gone to his supervisor, but now he took his problem to his peers, the surgical nurse practice group. They came up with a solution; the day nurse would fill out a form if she could not restock, and the evening nurses would put a note on the door if the room was not up to standards. Also the practice group would review all notes and counsel offenders if appropriate. As a result of their efforts, compliance improved.

According to Porter-O'Grady, during an interview for *OR Manager* (1988), shared governance gives staff nurses authority for decisions about their area of responsibility — nursing practice, education, and quality assurance. He points out that the traditional hospital system is not designed for nursing practice. Staff nurses have responsibility for performing duties assigned by others, and managers make the decisions and are held accountable. This conflict between the system's structure and nursing professionalism "drives the best nurses away from the bedside" (p. 1). The purpose of shared governance is to bring accountability and responsibility together. In this model authority is aligned with accountability (in other words, the person responsible has control of decision making) and autonomy is encouraged.

St. Joseph's Hospital in Atlanta, Georgia, which has more than eight years' experience with shared governance, organizes nurses within five councils: management, practice, education, quality assurance, and coordination (Porter-O'Grady, 1988). These councils have ultimate authority over their respective areas. They are comprised largely of staff nurses and are chaired by a staff nurse. Other members are a nurse manager, a clinical specialist, and a nurse administrator, who is an advisor without vote. The councils meet one day each month to address their areas of focus. In order to speed up responses to problems, a council chairperson can make a decision without input from other members; the decision is then reviewed at the next meeting.

Porter-O'Grady (1988) reports that time savings with this system have amounted to $25,000 at one hospital. Although this is not a large sum, it is evidence that the time the process takes is balanced by overall cost savings. Porter-O'Grady believes the savings are due to a decrease in short, fragmented, and nonproductive meetings and an increase in meetings that achieve their goal. Another benefit of shared governance is a decrease in turnover rate from 28 to 4 percent.

Shared Leadership. A major criticism of the shared-governance approach, according to Ericka Waidley (as cited in Anthony, 1990), is that it builds a power base for nurses at the expense of follow employees. This is one of the reasons John Gaffney, CEO at Irvine Medical Center (IMC) in California, chose not to use shared governance in the hospital's innovative process for administration: shared leadership. Shared leadership places decision-making authority at the point of patient-care delivery. The goals of the model are to satisfy customers (including physicians, patients, and hard-to-recruit professionals), to decrease bureaucracy and thereby increase action orientation, and to increase profitability. Rose Kennedy, of the IMC planning team, stresses, "You fill your hospital with leaders when you empower people to make decisions at the point of service. You energize the environment because people feel accountable for everything that takes place in the hospital" (as cited in Anthony, 1990, p. 1).

This radical approach eliminates middle management, the chief operating officer, the nursing director, supervisors, and head nurses. Their responsibilities are assigned to employees at the patient-care level who allot 10 to 40 percent of their time to administration as part of self-managed work teams. There are only nine mid-level managers. They act as coaches for their clusters of associated services. For example, a cluster in the Service Management Division includes support services such as social services, discharge planning, registration, chaplaincy, parking, and patient transportation.

The culture is in part defined by the elimination of terms such as *employee* and *committee;* these terms are replaced with *team members* and *issue action teams.* Issue action teams address shared concerns that involve more than one unit. These teams cover quality management, education, budgetary issues, in-service, relationships among units, and health care delivery. A team is composed of a volunteer member from each patient-care unit who serves for six months. In combination these employees function much as the traditional head nurse functioned. To add to the empowerment of staff, IMC teaches its team members to resolve conflicts and solve problems directly without supervisory intervention.

IMC's patient care is organized into three service lines: orthopedics, women's and children's services, and community medicine. These service lines are seen as independent businesses that contribute revenue to the hospital as a whole; they operate on a case-management model. The remaining parts of the organization — information services, shared services, service management, and physician services — focus on supporting the revenue-generating activities. They operate as efficient, low-cost vendors to the product lines.

IMC relies heavily on cross-training. It planned to have all staff cross-trained by the end of the fourth year. For example, a laboratory technician is able to fill in for a pharmacy technician to cover temporary vacancies. In addition, employees must spend a day each year handling someone else's job.

Other components of the participative style at IMC are the assignment of "buddies" to new employees to help them adjust to their new environment and the use of "brown-bag" sessions. These sessions are held to update employees on new policies or hospital trends. Team members rotate responsibility for conducting the sessions so each member gets an opportunity to supervise.

Employees are evaluated on both competence and service excellence. Credit is also given for participation in administration and planning. Eventually, employees will be evaluated by their own peers.

Because this process is still in its early stages, it is too soon to evaluate it. Gaffney, the CEO, admits that increases in productivity and profitability are not guaranteed. In addition, the hospital is still working out problems with productivity monitoring and management intervention in areas such as risk management and quality assurance. Also, because of Joint Commission on Accreditation of Healthcare Organizations standards UMC may need to make alterations in its nursing-administration line of command. Yet, IMC has added a bold innovation to health care, and administrators will be watching as this approach evolves.

Working as a Team

In summary, customers, including patients, employers, and payers, are demanding appropriate utilization of financial, social, psychological, technical, and medical resources by all care providers. It is no longer acceptable for clinical staff to be separated from the financial aspects of their patient's care. It is no longer acceptable for professionals to work independently of one another, duplicating and at times contradicting one another's work. It is no longer acceptable to claim turf at the expense of patient care.

In ancient Greece citizens prayed for the god Chaos to visit their village, for it was out of chaos that creation came. Patient-centered care is born of the chaos of modern times. This chaos is challenging us to examine our values, purpose, and mission. Health care is challenged to create new systems, new models, and new approaches to care. In general, the findings so far suggest that these models improve the interaction between team members as well as increase service to patients, the center of our care. Yet, we are early in the process; innovation is just beginning. New models will emerge, and some will be discarded. We are calling on professions and all caregivers to redefine their roles and their identities in the light of the formation of these new systems.

Chapter 6

Creating a Healing Environment

A hospital is no place for a person who is seriously ill.

Norman Cousins, *Anatomy of an Illness
as Perceived by the Patient**

As we examine patient-focused care, we become aware of the need to combine the "high tech" of the latest medical advancements with an environment that promotes "high touch," or personal interaction. In this chapter we will outline the impact that the environment can have on how individuals feel, as we explore some of the elements that constitute a healing environment. We will explain healing design principles and how to implement them in today's hospital. We will also explain how focusing on designing healing environments can enhance competitive advantage, and we describe key design principles for specific areas of the hospital as well as for specialized units.

Promoting Healing Through Design

At a symposium on health care–facility design, one consultant remarked that in all her years of designing health care environments, her clients would invariably mention functional requirements and stylistic preferences, but no one had ever asked her for an overall design for a healing environment. She believes that, in the not-too-distant future, designing such an environment may be the new frontier, and hospital administrators may expect their design consultants to know how to do it (Malkin,

*Norman Cousins, *Anatomy of an Illness as Perceived by the Patient,* © 1979 by W. W. Norton.

155

1991, p. 36). According to this consultant, perhaps one of the reasons environments that are conducive to healing are not emphasized is because we do not think of environments as having the potential to affect an individual's healing process. Also, since the early 1900s, the hospital has been designed as a functional and efficient medical workshop rather than as a center for integrating the power of the mind, spirit, and body to accelerate the healing process. The clean, sterile lines and lack of ornamentation that we associate with most modern hospitals have their roots in the modern architecture movement that began in Germany in the 1920s, which coincided with the beginning of high-tech scientific medicine. These buildings were designed to reflect the medical equivalent of the scientific model, with its values of objectivity, rationality, and efficiency.

In the past, the design of health care facilities emphasized efficiency and such functional factors as having doors wide enough to fit hospital beds. Unfortunately, design based on such functional concerns alone often ignores the psychological needs of patients, staff, and visitors and their need for warmth, comfort, and a nurturing environment. In an environment emphasizing functional efficiency, there is little consideration for the subjective experience of patients and the mystery and strong emotions associated with the drama that occurs in hospitals: birth, death, and dealing with illness.

The result is an environment that often has negative effects on both patients and staff. Specifically, research has shown that design that ignores basic psychological needs may actually lead to anxiety, elevated blood pressure, and an increase in the intake of pain-relieving drugs. Conversely, a warm, nurturing setting can induce a relaxation response and can therefore reduce medication levels and even decrease a patient's length of stay in the hospital (Ulrich, 1991).

It is ironic that we have designed hospitals with little attention to the elements that can enhance the healing process. In fact, Cousins (1979) found the hospital environment so noisy and disturbing that he decided to check himself into a hotel in order to recover from a near-fatal illness.

Adding Symbolic Meaning

Any environment is a mirror of the individual and of the culture. The environment reflects what individuals think about and feel and therefore echoes the values of the culture. An effective environment needs to be filled with cultural symbols that are meaningful, especially an environment aimed at healing. The absence of certain symbols indicates that members of the culture do not attach importance to certain ideas. For example, an environment that emphasizes the use of metallic surfaces sends the message that wood and other natural materials are not important. Because natural materials create a warm, homelike atmosphere, their absence reflects the lack of emphasis in the culture on that type of setting.

Symbols — or the lack of them — are significant in hospitals because patients come to hospitals to engage in life-changing events of great significance — the birth of children, the death of loved ones, and the healing of family members. Therefore, it makes sense for hospital architecture to reflect the symbolic role the hospital plays in the community. Yet most modern hospitals are not built with this role in mind. Hospitals are often plain, boxlike structures that hold no meaning and are not designed to convey the sacredness of their purpose. Perhaps the best way to describe what seems to be missing from the modern health care facility is to look at a "healing place" that existed before the modern hospital. In order to do that, let us journey back into time and explore the healing places of the past.

"These buildings seemed to organize shapes and powers, feelings and meanings into places that you could walk into and be tremendously moved" (Kellman, 1989, p. 20). The buildings referred to here are the hospitals of seventeenth- and eighteenth-century Europe. They had soaring vaulted ceilings, stained glass windows, artwork, and architectural ornamentation. In many ways, their design echoed that of Europe's great cathedrals because the presence of the sacred was integrated into the form of the buildings. In describing the buildings that served as hospitals in Europe over 500 years ago, Kellman has pinpointed the missing factor — a sense of place, a form appropriate to the mission of healing. The "healing cathedral" of the seventeenth and eighteenth century provided an uplifting, spiritual experience for patients, whereas the modern hospital seems to be merely a "body shop."

Another example from the past is the healing center of ancient Greece. People journeyed to these 300 to 400 healing centers in times of illness, crisis, or spiritual need. They remained at these temples for days or even weeks at a time. The sites for these ancient healing centers were carefully chosen. Location was thought to be crucial in determining the power of these environments to heal. The buildings were designed in harmony with their natural settings in order to draw on the healing power of nature and to emphasize the sacredness of the landscape.

The ancient Greeks understood the importance of an approach that integrated body, mind, and spirit. Patients at these centers engaged in a variety of activities in the libraries, theaters, gardens, gymnasiums, and baths. All these activities were designed to restore the body's rhythms and the harmony of the body and mind.

The power of the natural elements to aid in the healing process and the importance of restoring harmony between mind and body were central to the philosophy in these centers. All of them acknowledged the importance of place and the need for connection with the sacred.

Perhaps we moderns can learn from these ancient centers how to remake the hospital as a powerful symbol in our society; here, after all, is where the drama of life and death occurs. It is possible for the hospital of the future to again instill meaning and convey powerful messages about the natural life cycle and the potential of the healing process to be a journey of self-discovery.

The goal in designing a health care environment should be to provide a setting where form follows function. If the function of a hospital is to harness the healing potential of the whole human being, then we must create forms that echo this function. Therefore, it seems natural to say that the health care center of the future will be nothing like the hospital of today. As one futurist explains, the health care center of the future will use its specialized environment and architectural form to transmit a powerful message of healing. It will be a "high push" environment, one that is individualized and responsive to a patient's need for healing (McKahan, 1991, p. 4).

Reasons to Focus on Design

Perhaps the most important reason for creating the best possible hospital environment is the competitive advantage it gives to the institution. An article in *Hospitals Magazine* stated that to compete successfully in the 1990s, hospitals have to place a tremendous emphasis on design and architecture (cited in Malkin, 1991, p. 29).

Studies have shown that consumers evaluate health care organizations on the basis of such factors as the appearance of patient rooms and public spaces, the level of service, and the quality of interaction with caregivers. The "we care" message cannot stop with positive relationships and customer-service training. This message must be designed into the facility itself (Carpman, Grant, and Simmons, 1986, p. 11). The caring message and the dedication to quality service must be communicated from the moment the patient or visitor arrives at the facility.

Consumers who find their surroundings comforting and conducive to healing will be likely to return in the future and to recommend the hospital to friends and relatives. Because health care consumers have a choice about which providers they use, a superior environment that provides psychological and physical comfort can give a hospital a significant competitive advantage.

Creating a superior environment can also have a positive effect on staff satisfaction. A pleasant environment creates pride in being part of the organization and improves the well-being and mood of staff. Environment is important to all staff members, who are dependent on having adequate space for performing many different tasks, having appropriate lighting, and having a layout that allows for efficiently working with patients and coordinating the many services involved in patient care.

Design Considerations

Some of the most important considerations in designing health care environments are how to help patients and visitors find their way around the facility, how to provide physical comfort, how to regulate both social contact and privacy, and how to provide psychological comfort.

Effective Wayfinding Systems

Patient-centered care requires environments that are not only conducive to healing and attractive but also user-friendly. All users of hospital facilities, including patients, visitors, and staff, should be able to find their way around the various buildings quickly and easily. The environment must feel welcoming and accessible, rather than confusing and intimidating. Carpman, Grant, and Simmons's study (1986, p. 56) indicated that one of the greatest sources of stress for visitors was not being able to find their way around the hospital. Their confusion also has a negative effect on the attitude of patients because if their visitors spend time wandering around the hallways, lost and confused, the visitors may have less time to spend with them. For these reasons, it is crucial to ease the journey within the facility by implementing an efficient wayfinding system. Designers need to use a systematic approach for providing signs and directions both within the hospital and outside the facility.

A complete wayfinding system should consist of a variety of devices including informational signs, color coding, "you-are-here" maps, clearly marked floor levels, and major directional signs. Because wayfinding is such an integral part of a positive environment, we offer some general guidelines for effective wayfinding systems in three important areas: arrival at the facility, admissions, and circulation within the facility.

Arrival at Facility. Orientation devices located in an area where patients and their visitors first arrive need to focus on more than just the interior of the facility. Patients and visitors must be able to find their way from the parking lot to the correct department or building. The most important communication channel here is messages printed on interior and exterior signs. "You-are-here" maps need to be placed at the pedestrian exit from each parking area. These maps should be oriented so that forward is up (if the visitor is facing east, the map should be oriented so that east is at the top of the map). It is also important to place a set of maps and signs at the entrance to the facility. An information desk located near the entrance can be a source of additional directional information. Wording on signs should be consistent throughout the facility. Keep messages short, no more than seven words per sign. The best combination of colors for clarity on signs is black on yellow or black on white. It is also important that buildings be given understandable names that make sense to patients and visitors — for example, "general hospital" or "hospital" rather than "medical pavilion."

Admissions. The admissions department is usually the first destination for inpatients. Two design considerations here are that patients and their companions need a comfortable place to wait and a private place to talk. Patients need to have privacy in the admissions area because they report here a wide range of personal information. The best design for this area includes partitions or private offices. Also, wheelchair access is crucial. And patient records need to be stored in a place where confidentiality is ensured.

Circulation Within the Facility. Patients, visitors, and staff use the corridors, elevators, and stairways of a hospital to arrive at their destination and often spend time there waiting, getting information, and talking. Patients and visitors are usually under stress and filled with anxiety. For this reason, they are often too preoccupied to pay close attention to signs as they navigate the confusing, mazelike hallways of the facility. Therefore, it is important to assure that these signs are easy to understand. Also, often hospitals are large, complex facilities made up of many buildings that have been built over a period of time. Patients may have to visit several different locations within several buildings.

Here are some general guidelines for facilitating circulation within the hospital complex:

- Develop a comprehensive wayfinding system that includes interior and exterior landmarks, signs, maps, clear terminology, color coding, an easy-to-understand floor and room numbering system, and verbal directions.

- If possible, place services that are used by patients often in close proximity (admissions, laboratories, and x-ray rooms).
- Use interior landmarks such as lighting, color, texture, artwork, and plants to differentiate parts of the hospital. A similar appearance for all locations results in unnecessary confusion.
- Floor numbers should start on the main entrance floor and should indicate whether the floor is above or below ground level. Such a system is especially important for people using elevators.
- Design a floor numbering system that can be easily integrated into the room numbering system for each level.
- Design a room numbering system that is flexible enough to allow for future expansion and renovation.
- Place patient room numbers so they are visible when the door is open.
- If the health care facility has a large number of users for whom English is a second language, consider using multilingual signs.
- Because many technical and medical terms may not be understood by patients and visitors, use lay terms rather than medical terms for sections of the hospital. (In surveys, patients have stated that the ease of understanding terminology would influence their choice of a hospital [Carpman, Grant, and Simmons, 1986, p. 56].)
- Develop place names that are not confusing. Avoid terms like *child center,* which could be interpreted as a nursery or as a pediatric medical-care area.
- Use symbols or pictographs in conjunction with the verbal messages.
- Use colored lines on the floor along with other color wayfinding aids as part of an overall system. Color coding should be logical and consistent throughout the facility.
- Consider implementing an ongoing staff-training program for giving accurate directions; staff will continue to be asked for directions regardless of how good the wayfinding system is.

Physical Comfort

Patients, visitors, and staff perceive the hospital environment as comfortable based on factors such as temperature, noise levels, lighting, and odors.

Noise. When designing hospitals, it is important to pay attention to creating an environment that is restful. In this regard, the issue of noise must be addressed. Noise levels can be controlled in several ways. Sound-muffling material can be installed between patient rooms by using wall insulation. Within rooms, carpeting and other absorptive surfaces can alleviate this problem. Also, noisy activity areas like nurses' stations should be located away from patient rooms. Finally, staff should avoid holding conversations directly outside patient rooms.

Lighting. Lighting can influence hormonal secretions and can regulate circadian rhythms (Malkin, 1991, p. 35). One lighting-design consultant has stated that electric lighting and interior lighting in general can affect both physiological and psychological well-being. Light can be used to create nurturing, low-stress spaces that enhance a patient's recovery and improve attitude and well-being (Benya, 1989, p. 55). Therefore, attention needs to be paid to varying the types of lighting and the intensity of lighting in different areas of the hospital. One possibility is to have a flexible system of different light sources, each adjustable by multiple switches or a timer. Staff concerns include having adequate light for examining patients and night lights for nocturnal monitoring.

Patients and visitors need flexible lighting for various activities. For example, low lighting is needed for watching television, while task lighting is best for reading or writing, and medium-level lighting is best for conversation with several visitors. Therefore, room lighting needs to be adjustable, and controls should be within easy reach of patients and staff. A reading light should be close to the patient's bed, and a night light is needed to illuminate the path from bed to bathroom. Indirect lighting should also be provided so patients and visitors do not always need to have bright lights on.

Traditionally, health care facilities use cool-white or light-white fluorescent lamps and standard, inexpensive fixtures. With new advances in lighting design, health care facilities now have many options. These new options include softer lighting to reduce the harsh effect created by fluorescent lighting. Softer light can be created by using indirect lighting, wall washing, and task lighting.

Regulation of Social Contact and Privacy

Patients need both privacy and interaction with family and friends. Social support has been found to be a contributing factor in reducing stress and in accelerating the rate of recovery from illness (Carpman, Grant, and Simmons, 1986). Studies have shown that patients with high levels of social support experience less stress and have higher levels of general wellness. Those with lower levels of social support have slower recovery rates and higher rates of illness. The health benefits of high levels of social support have been well enough documented to justify planning health care facilities to encourage access to social support. The challenge is to provide patients with some degree of control so that they can balance social interaction and privacy.

Examples of amenities that increase social support are overnight accommodations for families of patients and comfortable visitor waiting areas with moveable seating, outdoor gardens, and sitting arrangements that encourage social interaction.

Privacy and the preservation of patients' dignity can be ensured in other ways. Admitting areas should have private offices, tall partitions, and spatial separation of task areas. Also, most patients find hospital gowns embarrassing and humiliating. Purchasing less revealing gowns or providing a robe shows respect for a patient's dignity. Patients are concerned too about whether they can be seen from the hallway. When given a choice, patients prefer to have the foot rather than the head of their bed positioned in line with the doorway (Carpman, Grant, and Simmons, 1986). Within rooms curtains provide visual access to and from patients' beds. To regulate their privacy, patients should have the ability to manipulate them.

Privacy in diagnostic and treatment rooms is also an important issue. One idea is to position the examining table so the patient is not exposed to people in the hallway when the door is open. Auditory privacy can be increased by constructing walls from the floor to the underside of the structural slab. Fully insulating this space with sound-muffling material can also be helpful.

Psychological Comfort

In order to meet the psychological needs of patients, consideration needs to be given to many different design elements to be sure that the messages they convey are meaningful to patients and help them to heal. These elements include lighting and ways to regulate privacy (which have been discussed), variety, color, artwork, and access to nature.

Variety. Variety in any environment is important, especially in a setting where individuals are likely to be stressed and anxious. Rather than providing a monotonous, sterile environment, a health care facility should use a variety of colors, textures, and fabrics. Distinctive landmarks such as artwork can also break up the sameness of a specific space.

Other elements can be used to create a comfortable, soothing setting. As mentioned, wood and other natural materials make a room seem homelike and welcoming. Carpeting also can humanize the health care environment. In addition, carpeting prevents the serious injuries that can result when patients fall. Carpeting needs to be stain resistant and must have a surface that minimizes the friction of wheeled equipment.

Color. Color can be used to create a mood, lift the spirit, or make a room appear cheerful. We have all experienced the negative effect of being in an environment that is drab. An imaginative application of color in a health care setting can be found in the buildings at the Vidarkliniken in Jarna, Sweden. Different areas of this facility are painted different colors so that a patient's stages of recovery can be matched to the best color by moving the patient from one area to another as recuperation progresses. For example, when patients are very ill, they are placed in a room with pale rose-colored walls. As they recover, the spaces they are moved into have more stimulating colors. This is one example of a conscious effort to tap the symbolic power of color to enhance the healing process.

Perhaps it is also time that we in the United States rethink our allegiance to the traditional hospital white. Color can be used to brighten a space and add warmth and a feeling of comfort. Color can also be added to the hospital environment through artwork, murals on the walls, and in sheets, gowns, bedspreads, accessories, and even food trays.

Integrating Artwork. Art can be used to make a space attractive while providing much-needed distraction from worried thoughts or the experience of pain. Photographs or pictures of scenes of nature can hold a patient's attention and can also block stressful thoughts, which increase anxiety levels. It is especially important to have artwork in patient rooms and waiting areas. These spaces must provide enough stimulation to counteract boredom, depression, and anxiety.

Research on artwork preference indicates that patients enjoy artwork that depicts natural subjects and prefer representation over abstraction. Participants in a number of empirical studies consistently preferred photographs of natural views dominated by vegetation or water to views of urban scenes (Carpman, Grant, and Simmons, 1986, p. 197). The images found to be the most pleasing were those that were far removed from a patient's current situation, such as natural, beautiful, peaceful scenes (p. 171).

Providing Access to Nature. Views of nature can also promote positive feelings, reduce negative emotions, and hold attention, thus effectively blocking stressful or worried thoughts (Ulrich, 1991, p. 103). Visual contact with nature even for as short a time as ten minutes can help in reducing stress. Research indicates that views of nature produce a more rapid and complete reduction of stress than do views of urban scenes (p. 103).

Nature in health care–facility design can be integrated in several ways. Views from windows are important so that all patients, especially long-term, critically ill patients, can feel connected with the outside world. Nature can also be brought into the interior space of the hospital by including skylights and atriums. Plants can be integrated into the hospital space by providing planters and window boxes in rooms. Although plants are not appropriate for all hospital environments, specifically not for surgical suites and recovery rooms, they can be soothing and healing for patients and visitors in other areas.

Paying attention to the design of outdoor spaces is just as important as finding ways to bring the outdoors in. Some of the guidelines to follow in designing these spaces include planting as many trees as possible, providing a variety of seating arrangements, and arranging design elements so that patients, families, and visitors have a sense of privacy.

Putting It All Together: Mid-Columbia Medical Center

As we examine the components of a healing environment, it may be helpful to examine one hospital that has remodeled its facility to integrate many of these elements. That facility is Mid-Columbia Medical Center in The Dalles, Oregon. Mid-Columbia based its remodeling on the ideas developed at Planetree (San Francisco) in order to create a homelike, nurturing environment.

The goals of the renovation project included upgrading areas of the hospital that had not been touched since they were first built and redesigning parts of the hospital to be more user-friendly. The project included renovating or adding activity rooms, solariums, family dining areas, and an atrium, and making patient rooms more pleasant.

Some of the specific changes included renovating patient rooms by adding or upgrading window treatments, flooring, paint, wallpaper, closets, and lighting. Each patient room is now also equipped with a television set and an audiocassette recorder. Sleeper chairs have been installed to accommodate family members. Shelves have been hung in each room so that patients can place their flowers and personal belongings on them.

In addition, newly designed activity rooms on two patient floors provide a comfortable place where patients and visitors can talk, read, relax, or watch movies. An atrium was added to create a beautiful new entrance and provide a natural and peaceful environment for patients, families, and friends.

Following the model of Planetree, Mid-Columbia replaced the traditional nurses' station with an open work station and patient-resource area. This new design encourages interaction between patients and the nursing staff.

As in the Planetree unit, patient education is integral to the philosophy at Mid-Columbia. There are libraries on the patient floors where patients and family members can obtain information and read about the treatment of diseases.

The existing staff kitchens on patient floors were expanded into kitchen/dining areas. Kitchens are now used by family members to prepare home-cooked meals. Dieticians also use the kitchens and plan programs that teach patients about nutrition.

Art and entertainment are other important elements at Mid-Columbia. Patients have access to audiocassette players and a wide variety of music. A movie night allows patients, families, and friends to watch a movie together. Entertainers, including storytellers and musicians, regularly visit the facility. The paintings on the walls of patient rooms and hallways have been carefully selected to enhance the aesthetic quality of the environment.

Design Principles for Specific Areas

Design principles for specific areas of the hospital integrate the elements we have covered so far, but some concepts apply to only one area. We will review these ideas in this section by looking at waiting areas, patient rooms, and diagnostic/examination areas.

Waiting and Reception Areas

Waiting is part of the hospital experience for both patients and visitors. Waiting may occur in patient rooms, in hallways, in clinics, in lobbies, and in reception areas. Although waiting in itself is often a negative experience, the design of waiting and reception areas can alleviate some of the negative aspects of this experience.

Here are some general guidelines for waiting and reception areas:

- Provide information about the location of restrooms, telephones, vending machines, and cafeterias.
- Include brochures about procedures and directions for going through the registration process. Research indicates that patients who have access to information about the admissions process are able to rely more on signs and are generally more satisfied with their hospital experience than are patients who do not have such information (Carpman, Grant, and Simmons, 1986, pp. 106–122).
- Make waiting rooms the right size — not too crowded for the average volume and also not so large that individuals feel lost or isolated.
- Locate waiting areas near major circulation paths, not in some obscure corner.
- Provide for a variety of activities — reading, watching television, playing with children, or simply sitting in solitude. Consider using dividers, alcoves, or plants to separate these activities.
- Provide a glass wall between the waiting area and the hall if possible. Visitors prefer to be able to see activities in the hall (Carpman, Grant, and Simmons, 1986).
- Provide seating for individuals, small groups, and large groups. People should be able to position themselves comfortably for conversation. Moveable furniture allows visitors to create their own seating arrangements.
- Consider ways to accommodate children by creating a play area located away from the circulation flow of the room.
- Provide a place for storage of personal belongings.
- Provide telephones.
- Make public restrooms accessible from hallways rather than through waiting areas.
- Provide vending machines close to waiting areas and stock them with nutritious foods.

Diagnostic and Treatment Areas

Patients on their way to treatment centers are usually in a state of fear: fear of procedures that are unfamiliar and often threatening, fear of the equipment used, fear of disease, and general fear of the unknown. The goal in this area needs to be to humanize the environment and reduce the stress of undergoing medical procedures. Here are some suggestions for designing treatment and diagnostic areas to alleviate stress and fear:

- Provide the maximum amount of privacy for patients by having lockable doors or curtains for the changing rooms.
- Locate the path from dressing room to gowned waiting and examination or treatment rooms out of public view.
- Keep dressing rooms slightly warmer than the rest of the facility.
- In dressing rooms, provide carpeting and comfortable chairs, and install hooks and shelves. Pleasant things to look at such as artwork and a mirror for grooming are also helpful.
- It helps if shiny equipment can be completely or partially concealed. In this way it is less intimidating to patients.
- Provide indirect, soft lighting in rooms where stressful procedures occur.

Patient Rooms

Because patients spend most of their time in their rooms, it is important to consider designing this space for maximum comfort and ease of communication with caregivers.

Privacy Needs. One of the crucial issues is providing privacy in patient rooms, especially rooms that are semiprivate. Patients also need to be able to control their privacy. For example, many patients like having an interior window so that they can watch activity in the hall. For staff, this window can also facilitate monitoring of patients. However, patients are also concerned about unwanted exposure through these windows. Therefore, it is important that curtains can be controlled by patients. This ability to regulate visual access allows patients a sense of autonomy.

Because auditory privacy is also important, there needs to be a clear division of territory for visitors for each patient in side-by-side semiprivate rooms.

A Room with a View. Views of the outside are important

for patients; windows give patients contact with the outside world and enable them to keep track of the seasons and the passage of time. If the view is pleasant, particularly if it is of a nature setting, it may even have therapeutic benefits. In general, windows should be as large as possible; they should provide views of activity at street level; they should be positioned near enough to the floor so wheelchair-bound patients can have a maximum view; and window coverings should be easily controlled by patients. A room should have photographs, pictures, and wall murals of nature views when actual nature views are not available.

Design Principles for Specialized Units

In this section we examine how to design specialized units by suggesting basic guidelines for the following spaces: physical rehabilitation centers, pediatric centers, hospices, and birthing facilities.

Physical Rehabilitation Centers

According to design experts who plan rehabilitation facilities, one of the primary considerations is providing a space that motivates patients who are involved in an often intensely personal, long-term physical and psychological process (Guynes, 1990, p. 37). The space must be designed to motivate a patient to come every day despite the pain and often the embarrassment involved in rehabilitation therapy. The importance of a suitable environment for rehabilitation centers is expressed by one designer, who states that the environment truly affects a patient's rate of healing. In rehabilitation, the environment can motivate patients to do the hard work necessary for recovery and can convince them that they can become functional again (Guynes, 1990, p. 39).

In addition to patient motivation, a rehabilitation center must also promote staff well-being and motivation. Rehabilitation-center staff are usually under tremendous psychological pressure because their patients not only are physically disabled but often are depressed.

Traditionally, not much attention has been paid to the

design of rehabilitation areas. Usually rehabilitation centers end up in the basement of the hospital in a space that encourages neither patient motivation nor staff satisfaction. Now, however, because of the growing importance of rehabilitation therapy, rehabilitation areas are being given increased attention.

Rehabilitation today focuses on helping patients perform daily tasks and become functional in the outside world. Therefore, it is important to design rehabilitation spaces where patients can practice skills such as getting in and out of a car. In addition, rehabilitation areas must provide space for equipment; be able to accommodate varying case loads; meet safety regulations; and provide space for staffing, charting, admitting, and clerical activities.

In designing rehabilitation units, it is important to obtain input from the therapy staff, the head of the rehabilitation department, and the hospital administrator. Physicians' input is, needless to say, also crucial because physicians are the source of referrals for rehabilitation units.

Pediatric Facilities

As we examine the importance of environment in health care facilities and how it can affect feelings and behavior, it probably comes as no surprise that environment is particularly important in facilities for children. Research has shown that children remember places and sensations more than they remember people. Therefore, design must take into account a child's acute sensitivity to physical surroundings (Hall, 1990, p. 65). Whether the facility is a children's hospital or a pediatric unit in a general hospital, it is important to focus on children's special needs and how these can be integrated into the design.

Accommodating Parents. One of the most important aspects of designing an environment for children is to recognize the need to accommodate parents and other family members. Many hospitals, for example, have a twenty-four-hour visiting policy, which allows parents to room-in with their child. Some amenities that need to be included are extra beds, showers, storage areas, and lounges where parents can relax and interact with other parents.

Parents often stay with their children during anesthesia induction and recovery or during tests or emergency procedures; they need to be able to do so in a space separate from the sterile area of the surgical suite. Being able to stay with a child is especially important for parents of children in ICUs, where adequate accommodations are not common. One design idea is to provide rooms near the ICU for parents to sleep in.

Providing for privacy is essential when designing spaces that need to accommodate children and their families. Family members must be able to choose the level of privacy needed. Attention needs to be paid to seating and how it is arranged and whether it promotes or inhibits interaction with others. For example, creating privacy zones in the ICU is one idea. These zones may be a corner with a sofa, a plant, and a view where both parents and staff can relax.

Designing for Children. From the moment children enter the facility, they should feel welcome. The environment should be appealing to all children from the very young infant to the young adult. One way to make a space inviting to children is by including graphics. For example, children's drawings can be painted on novel surfaces such as tiles.

Because play is so fundamental an activity for children, it is important to have play areas and playrooms throughout the facility. Children also enjoy interacting with their environment so including design elements that invite participation can be an interesting idea. Children might be allowed to decorate their rooms or personalize their environment in other ways. Rooms can include surfaces on which children can display cards and drawings or chalkboards on which children can draw or write. The new Children's Hospital of Jacksonville (Florida) has an interactive wall with books, gadgets, toys, and medical exhibits. By manipulating knobs on this wall, children can turn x-ray pictures on and off, assemble medical models, and explore the human senses. The environment should also provide the potential for interaction by including interesting objects to look at and spaces to respond to and explore. Because children learn through movement, children need to be able to move about freely in these spaces.

Another important consideration in designing health care

environments for children is the need to preserve the spirit of the child in the design features. One designer has described this spirit as "a sense of wonder, . . . a sense of openness, trust and responsiveness, an ability to be" (Olds, 1991, p. 111). In line with this spirit of openness, an interesting idea is designing around the "aesthetic richness" of a space. In doing so, we transcend our conventional conception about a room so that any surface can be a toy, a seat, a wall, or a divider (p. 112).

Including the presence of nature is especially crucial in designing facilities for children. Bringing the outdoors in can be accomplished by including plants, pools of water, fountains, and views of the outdoors. Outdoor space should include both play areas and seating areas.

Another design consideration, which is equally applicable for adult facilities, is providing distractions from the fear-provoking equipment in treatment areas. For example, one radiology treatment room at a children's hospital is decorated with murals and mobiles that can keep children's attention while they are undergoing treatment. At one children's hospital, children come to a preoperative playroom thirty minutes before sedation. This room is like a big living room. It has a play frame, a platform with objects that can be manipulated, and a raised bench for older children. Often families and children wait in this room, where they can play together or talk. Doctors come into this room to discuss procedures with the parents in an environment that is much more conducive to these types of conversation than an office.

An example of a space specifically designed for children is the Starbright Pavilion in Los Angeles (Starbright Pavilion Foundation, 1992). The entry plaza is filled with giant toys. Inside, a "yellow brick road" lights up when you walk in. An atrium is a five-level "kids' town" of storefronts and includes spaces where children can climb and play. There are also a scaled-down trolley car and a theater where children can watch movies, television, and live performances.

In summary, pediatric units or other spaces for children should be designed with the spirit of playfulness that all children have. In order to help alleviate the anxiety of both children and their parents, the environment must be welcoming, home-like, and cheerful.

Birthing Units

Creating birthing units that are functional and have a strong appeal to women can give the hospital an important competitive edge. One of the reasons that responding to the needs and wants of women is so important is that research has shown that women make the majority of health care decisions for both themselves and their families (Vogler, 1990, p. 121). If a woman has had a positive experience at a particular hospital, she and her family will most likely return (Vogler, 1990, p. 125). As a result, hospitals have begun to design birthing environments that are sensitive to the wishes of these potential customers (Vogler, 1990, p. 121).

Because women are having fewer children, each birth is very special. Women want a caring, dignified environment for this event. For this reason, hospitals need to be aware of the elements that make one facility different from others. Unique touches, such as VCRs or sleep sofas for fathers, can make a substantial difference in successfully marketing birthing facilities.

Design Elements. Designing birthing areas requires creating comfortable homelike settings where women can be treated with dignity and have their needs met. Perhaps the biggest change affecting birthing-space design is the move from a multiple transfer system, in which a woman is wheeled from a labor room to a delivery room and then to a recovery room, to single-room maternity care. In the single-room model, a woman remains in one area for all four steps of the birthing process — labor, delivery, recovery, and postpartum. Some hospitals have a modified approach, which involves one move after delivery into a separate postpartum room (Vogler, 1990).

Research indicates that from a continuity-of-care perspective, the single-room model is preferable; however, from a practical perspective, one is not preferable to the other. The decision to use one or the other usually depends on space availability.

According to experts who have designed birthing areas,

some important clinical considerations must be addressed (Vogler, 1990, p. 124). The room should be at least 350 square feet, and the narrowest part should be at least 14 feet so that staff members have room to function. Equipment in the room must not block access to the patient. It is also important to provide enough electrical outlets and storage areas for equipment.

Surveying Nurses. One of the best ways to start designing birthing facilities is to survey target groups in order to determine what is important to them. These groups may include nurses, women consumers, and physicians. For nurses, single-room maternity care is attractive. This type of setting provides them with opportunities to use additional professional skills because they must be cross-trained in several nursing disciplines in order to work in single-room maternity areas. Therefore, if a hospital wants to attract well-qualified nurses and keep them motivated, such facilities are essential.

Hospices

A hospice is based on the concept that death is a natural part of life and that people need a special environment as they near the end of their journey. The purpose of a hospice is to relieve physical suffering and offer a place that is supportive to both patients and their families. The National Hospice Organization defines a hospice as a "medically directed multi-disciplinary program providing skilled care . . . for terminally ill patients and their families to live as fully as possible until the time of death" (quoted in Gappell, 1990, p. 77).

The environment of the hospice can affect the quality of the process of dying for both patients and their families. The hospice needs to provide contact with nature and encourage spirituality. It needs to allow patients to find meaning, review their life, and, finally, to accept death. The design of the hospice must also respond to the needs of caregivers and must allow family members to share their feelings and express their grief. The death of a loved one is one of the highest stressors in life (Gappell, 1990, p. 77). For this reason, the hospice environment must emphasize relaxation and allow for privacy.

Hospice rooms must include access to nature and sunlight. A hospice facility should have as much natural light as possible from windows and skylights. Electrical fixtures should use bulbs that have a color similar to daylight. All light should be soft and nonglaring to reduce stress.

Color is another important consideration because different colors have different effects on individuals. Colors can stimulate and excite, or they can soothe and heal. Blue, for example, increases relaxation and decreases anxiety. Warm, soft colors like peach and violet can produce feelings of comfort. Some of the colors and color combinations to be avoided are yellow tones, which are associated with the color of body fluids, and dramatic color contrasts, which can be tiring.

Because noise is a major source of stress, controlling noise is important in hospice facilities. Studies reveal that patients require more pain medication when noise levels are increased (Gappell, 1990, p. 78). One way to reduce noise is to use carpeting and soft materials for curtains and wall coverings.

Music also lowers stress and anxiety. Research has shown that music can alter moods and have a soothing effect (Gappell, 1990). Having a music library in a hospice is an excellent idea.

Additional elements that should be included in hospice facilities are larger bedrooms than those in traditional facilities, overnight accommodations for families, family gathering space, artwork that depicts nature scenes, and kitchenettes.

Choosing Design Teams

As health care facilities examine their needs for new structures or remodeling, they need to develop criteria for selecting designers. The two words that seem to come up again and again are *quality* and *relationship*. As one client of a design company stated, "The quality of the work done directly relates to the quality of the relationship developed between the health care provider and designer" (Ambers, Boyd, and Ray, 1991, p. 54). Because this relationship is so important, designers should be involved early in the process, as soon as the basic plan is defined. Designers should be involved at the same time as architects.

Some of the factors to consider when choosing designers, such as longevity and reputation, are obvious. It is also crucial that the designers be committed to conducting their own research on the latest trends in health care design and the types of facilities most hospitals are building. For example, the four major specialty areas of health care that will grow in the future are women's and children's facilities, heart care, cancer care, and rehabilitation services (Ambers, Boyd, and Ray, 1991, p. 54). A design team that conducts its own market research to discover pertinent facts such as this will have a great deal of relevant information to bring to the planning and design of these facilities.

In addition, designers should be customer-oriented enough to gather information about their clients, including understanding the culture of the organization and learning what is important to the client and how to satisfy the needs of patients, visitors, and staff. Successful design schemes focus in particular on the needs of the patient. Involving patients in choosing color schemes and fabrics is one way to be patient-focused.

Getting input from many groups is important; however, designers also must be able to communicate their own recommendations in a direct manner. For example, designers are final experts on color and should therefore be assertive rather than merely saying what the clients want to hear when decisions about color are being made. When designers receive information from several user groups such as patients and staff, they should not attempt to please the most vocal group but rather should integrate all viewpoints and be able to offer clear and rational explanations for their design recommendations (Ambers, Boyd, and Ray, 1991, p. 57).

In addition, it is important to choose designers who have a broad view of the project and who consider the entire complex by aiming at consistency. Although this may seem to be an obvious rule of good design, some designers get carried away by a new direction and do not pay attention to the need for unity in the overall design scheme.

Good designers also have detailed knowledge of finishes and materials. They should research the latest trends and know whether new materials are superior to already existing materials.

Because health care providers are always concerned about present and future costs, it is important too for designers to be aware of the maintenance and upkeep required for the materials they recommend using. Being sensitive to cost differences is always important. Designers need to know when to save money and when a more expensive choice is necessary to create a specific effect.

Perhaps the most important aspect is the need for designers to understand the needs of the specific patient population that the facility is being designed for. Designing a birthing center is obviously different from designing rooms for long-term-care patients.

Redesigning the Health Care Environment

Today's patient-focused consumer wants both the best in medical technology and personal attention provided within a warm, nurturing environment. We need to be especially sensitive to how much the physical environment affects a patient's mind and emotions. In this chapter we have explored some of the components of a healing environment.

As we move away from the traditional hospital environment to a sensory-rich, multidimensional environment that nurtures the whole person, we are redefining the very nature of the hospital. These new spaces combine art, education, nature, light, and symbols to harness the healing potential inherent in all human beings. In the process of designing such spaces, we are rediscovering and reconnecting with a tradition that goes back to the great healing temples of ancient Greece, where healing was defined by restoring the balance of mind, body, and spirit. By implementing the design principles outlined in this chapter, our hospitals can become temples of healing, where form follows function and the sacred art of healing joins with the modern miracle of medical technology.

Chapter 7

Strategies for Implementing Healing Health Care

It is hard to get people in the hospital to understand they have to heal themselves before they can heal others.

Elisabeth Kübler-Ross, 1992

Restructuring services around the needs of patients is one aspect of patient-focused care; another aspect is how to provide those services in order to enhance patient and family healing. Healing, defined as wholeness and integration, is, at its core, about relationships. Because relationships exist both within the person and between people, there are both an internal and an external environment to consider in health care that heals as well as cures. In this chapter, we offer strategies for implementing a healing environment. We begin by exploring how an organization can develop therapeutic presence by offering supportive programs for the care providers. Next, we focus on patient and family empowerment, as we offer strategies that encourage active patient and family participation and learning. Then, we turn to strategies for implementing nontraditional therapies. We close this chapter with a review of commonly encountered barriers to organizational change efforts and share our learnings on how to overcome these barriers.

Therapeutic Presence

We in health care provide a human service; our product is produced and consumed simultaneously. Health care exists essentially in its people. At a workshop on life, death, and transition,

I (Nancy Moore) approached Elisabeth Kübler-Ross, who is credited with humanizing the dying process, asking for guidance. She replied, "You [the care givers] must heal yourselves. Everything else will follow quite naturally if you support the staff in their own healing." This section offers strategies for promoting the healing and growth of staff members. Only with this kind of support can caregivers be therapeutically present for patients.

Culture Building

Culture can be defined as the consciousness of the organization. The culture of the organization is reflected in everything that is the organization. The organization, from a systems point of view, is a living organism in and of itself. It has physical, mental, emotional, and spiritual aspects. The organization's culture is composed of and is a part of its larger community. The culture of the organization is enriched when there is a conscious intention to develop the organization's unique mythology. Kaiser (1991e) uses the term *mythology* in the sense of developing meaning: "A myth confers purpose or meaning upon the members of an organization. A spiritual organization can use the power of the myth to create a sense of 'presence' in the institution. A myth empowers people to act. . . . Ritual, ceremony, and celebration are necessary to maintain the power of myth. Each new person coming into the organization must be initiated into its history, traditions, and mythology. Without the living spirit, the forms are dead" (message 203). By using the following ideas, hospitals can develop a healing culture and mythology.

First, weave healing for the caregiver and patients into the fabric of the organization. For example, Sister Kathryn Hellman of St. Charles Medical Center offers a "Mission Alive" program that explores the healing mission and values of the hospital. Participants from all areas of the hospital join in small groups to explore their personal mission and values as they relate to the hospital's mission and values.

Second, utilize the community's mythology as a source for the hospital's healing ministry. For example, some hospitals in Hawaii use their rich mythology by offering classes for employees in "mana training." These classes help employees learn how to open themselves to mana (spiritual energy). St. Charles uses the hospital's logo, the fleur-de-lis, as a discussion point. Sister Kathryn explains how the horizontal dimension represents the material aspects of life and the vertical dimension represents the spiritual, a reminder of the need for inclusion of the spiritual in our healing work. Tucson Medical Center (TMC) of Tucson, Arizona, uses the rich mythology of the Native American traditions. Virginia Throssell, account executive for the government sector, says, "Making sure the tribe gets the service they want and need is close to my heart." Throssell arranges for discharge planners to visit the Tohono O'odham reservation so they will understand how to meet their people's needs. During these visits staff learn that Native Americans consider it impolite to ask questions or to indicate when they do not understand instructions. As a result, staff members are taught to check understanding by asking for specifics — for example, "Show me how you will feed the baby." Also, TMC goes the extra mile to make sure the Tohono O'odham people are supported in their traditions. Every effort is made to assure that Native American patients know they can have their traditional food brought in or have their doctor (medicine man) visit.

Third, offer retreats that include the subjective dimensions of caring and healing. These retreats can help rekindle the commitment that attracted caregivers to the helping professions in the first place. Retreats can be used also as a time to refresh and revitalize team members. New visions can be created, problems resolved, and action plans for improvement initiated.

Fourth, use art as a powerful conveyor of meaning. Sister Kathryn of St. Charles Medical Center sees art as a means of enabling people to come in harmony with the richness of the mind and the spirit as well as of the body. As a result of this belief in the power of art, St. Charles commissioned a sculptor, David Kocka, to create a symbol of compassion. After visiting and getting to know the people and community of St. Charles he created "The Yoke of Compassion." The hospital uses this art form as a discussion point for exploring the role of compassion and the mutual nature of healing. Sister Kathryn views this sculpture as a symbol for "enabling the healer to continue being open to receive from those being healed the gift of life that they have to give." During discussions staff are facilitated in exploring how patients have helped them in their own growth and healing as they were helping the patients.

Fifth, make the culture of the organization conscious and intentional. Lussier, CEO of St. Charles, facilitates a small group charged with defining and developing the hospital's culture. They began the process by looking at four areas: heritage, standards, symbols, and programs. Each of these areas was addressed by specific groups: patients, managers, employees, and physicians. For example, each group explored the hospital's heritage by answering these questions: What do we want to keep and take forward? What do we want to leave behind or change? Also, the same process was used in identifying clear standards and developing symbols and programs that support the culture. These decisions may be reflected in how people are selected, oriented, and trained; how decisions are made; how people communicate and care for one another; and how accomplishments are recognized. All these elements of an organization's culture can be described in orientation sessions, ongoing discussion groups, and employee newsletters, or printed on personal cards as reminders.

Staff Education About Healing

How many hospitals have classes on healing, or for that matter even use the word in their staff-development plan? I have not done a poll, but I feel comfortable in saying that there are not many. Yet, is healing not the business of health care? Much of the burn-out we experience in health care today is related to the emphasis on technological cure. When the emphasis is on curing alone, care providers cannot help but feel a sense of failure when death and illness take their toll regardless of their efforts. As a society we have been in denial that death and illness are a part of life. Acceptance of death and illness begins when we put the emphasis on healing as well as curing for both patients and caregivers. For example, at a workshop on team development at St. Charles Medical Center, where sessions on therapeutic presence, healing, and compassion were offered as part of the curriculum, a participant explained her own experience as a patient: "I felt like a nonperson. When I was sick, people avoided me and seemed uncomfortable around me. It made a huge difference who cared for me. Some nurses never asked me how I was feeling, and when I brought up my fears, they always seemed to leave the room. Other nurses were very comfortable in being with me and helping me explore my feelings. It made all the difference."

The following are topics to consider in offering caregiver education on healing:

1. Explore the meaning of the word *healing* and its relationship to curing.
2. Have staff members share their personal experiences with illness and healing.
3. Explore the concept of the wounded healer—that is, how staff members' own illnesses or injuries have helped them grow or helped them help others.
4. Explore how healing is reciprocal—for example, how patients have helped in the caregiver's healing.
5. Offer exercises that help caregivers experience a patient's point of view. For example, Mid-Columbia Medical Center uses an exercise called Blind Man's Walk. During this exercise participants break into two groups; one group is the caregiver, and the other group is the patient. The caregivers must remain silent while leading the blindfolded patients. Both groups then share their experiences from their point of view.
6. Offer a series of workshops for caregivers that focuses on developing basic counseling skills.

Employee Wellness

Hospital work is stressful. Caring for acutely ill and dying patients requires a great deal of personal giving and energy. I find it helpful to recall that there is little difference between the caregiver and the patient. They are both people with similar stresses and challenges of living. Another way to view the importance of caring for the caregiver is that as hospitals take on responsibility for healing their communities, they will become aware of the effect that healthier, happier employees and their families have in enriching community health. In addition, an axiom in health care is that you cannot give what you do not have. When employees are stressed out, sick, angry, or feeling unsupported, they cannot help patients to feel differently.

As a result, some hospitals have created wellness programs for their employees, including programs on stress management, exercise, and nutrition. St. Charles Medical Center utilized a consultant, Harry Owens, Jr., M.D., MIM, to develop personal and organizational programs for stress, wellness, and creativity. Another important approach for meeting this need is employee-assistance programs. These programs may be formal, or, as at California Pacific Medical Center, a psychiatric nurse practitioner may meet with staff members as needed on a weekly basis. These programs provide short-term counseling for employees and sometimes for their family members. A key component is alcohol and drug counseling. Many organizations, within and outside of health care, have found that employee assistance programs are cost-effective in that they decrease the use of sick time and enhance employee productivity.

Personal and Relational Growth Courses

The philosophy of TQM recognizes that people require more than money. They want ever-broadening opportunities to enrich society. Abraham Maslow (1968), pioneer in motivational theory, reminds us that after physiological and safety needs are met, people are motivated by social, self-esteem, and self-actualization needs. In health care, where our product is our people, it makes good sense to institute programs and support for personal and relational as well as professional growth.

Unfortunately, a great deal of hospital employees' time and energy goes into handling relationship problems with other staff members, physicians, and/or management. Too often these relationship problems are not openly acknowledged or addressed.

As a result, much employee and management time is spent either avoiding these issues or discussing them with everyone except those involved. For example, it is not uncommon to hear a manager say, "Oh I can't assign so and so with him. They don't like to work with each other." Yet there is no similar hesitation in fixing a piece of hospital equipment when it breaks down. We would not tolerate doing a CAT scan with a broken scanner or knowingly do radiation therapy with a poorly calibrated machine. Hospitals need to develop the same concern for the proper functioning of their people and relationships as for the proper functioning of equipment.

Being aware of this need, Washoe Medical Center of Reno, Nevada; Sutter Medical Center of Sacramento, California; and St. Charles Medical Center of Bend, Oregon, instituted personal and relational growth seminars for their employees. Bill Adamski, founder of the ART of Living Institute located in Sacramento, California, offers an intensive three-day course that focuses on helping participants practice the ontological discipline known as the ART Works Paradigm: "Acceptance of what is, responsibility for the experience of what is, trust in the ability of one's self and others to make appropriate choices in the face of what is."

This course as well as other personal and relational growth seminars, such as "Bringing Self to Work: Creating People-Focused Teams" by Leadership Dynamics of Eugene, Oregon, have contributed to improved productivity, commitment, and accountability and have enhanced team and personal communication. An added bonus has been the implementation of innovative programs as a result of participants' becoming more aligned with their vision and personal commitments. For example, Pam Higgins, graduate of and now a facilitator for the ART of Living Institute, created the "Healing Power of Grief" groups in Reno, Nevada. These groups are a tremendous community resource.

An important part of any ongoing personal-development program is follow-up and support. Hospitals have found that meeting on at least a monthly basis helps keep people on track with their commitments and learnings.

Critical Incident Debriefing

Hand in hand with support of employee wellness is critical-incident stress debriefing (CISD). Unfortunately, until relatively recently hospital personnel have silently endured extremes of stress without relief. The pressures of their jobs have negative effects on some employees, especially in acute-care areas, where tragedy is a common event. For these employees disruption in health and happiness takes the form of chronic sleep disturbance and distressing dreams and memories. These changes may lead to depression, anxiety, and anger. Healthy, committed people may begin hospital work only to leave it prematurely as a result of these stresses. Such premature loss of personnel or disruptions in their health and happiness are frequently preventable. Through the use of CISD significant stress reactions can be prevented or lessened.

The formal CISD process, lasting about three hours, is best performed after twenty-four hours and before seventy-two hours following a critical incident. It is led by a mental health professional and peer support personnel. There are an introduction phase, a fact phase, a thought phase, a reaction phase, a symptom phase, a teaching phase, a reentry phase, and post-debriefing activities. Also included are follow-up services and individual consultations as needed.

St. Charles is now extending this service to other area hospitals and key services in the community such as emergency medical services, police, schools, and mental health services. St. Charles plans to pool resources and training with these groups so that they can all serve as resources for one another. Readers are referred to Mitchell and Bray (1990), *Emergency Services Stress,* for a detailed description of this important way of enhancing the healing environment.

Team Development

Individuals are unlikely to succeed at enhancing healing, even when they work extraordinarily hard, unless they are part of a supportive team. The common threads of successful teams are a leadership style that emphasizes participation, facilitation, and coaching; a common vision with values and standards that are continuously reviewed; an ongoing emphasis on team maintenance, which includes personal and team accountability; and an emphasis on continuous improvement.

These strategies create the space and support for caregivers to be therapeutically present for their patients. If therapeutic presence is part of a hospital's philosophy, hiring people who share that philosophy and vision is important. To do so, the hospital's vision, values, and standards need to be clearly articulated during the hiring process. Hospitals owe it to themselves and those they employ to be clear about expectations before a job is taken. At Planetree nurses are chosen on the basis of their technical expertise and their ability to nurture, support, teach, and empower. At St. Charles, therapeutic presence is part of caregivers' position descriptions.

Patient and Family Empowerment

At first glance we may assume the active involvement of patients and families in care. Patients are probably spending at least $1,000 per day. Of course, they are active participants in their care. Of course, they are the focus of care. Of course, they are provided with access to all their test results and given all the information they desire about their illness and treatment. Yet, as any organization that begins to implement a patient-focused philosophy soon discovers, this is not the case.

Mark Scott, president of Mid-Columbia Medical Center (Oregon), a forty-nine-bed tertiary referral center that has implemented the Planetree model hospitalwide, relates that it took four and a half years to do it. According to Scott, "It began with a realization that what we are doing is not right. The typical hospital experience is intimidating, cold, and depersonalizing. Patients are treated like widgets instead of people. For me personally, if we couldn't do it differently, I was ready to leave it behind." Under the guidance of Planetree's national director of hospital projects, Scott set out to personalize, demystify, and humanize care.

New York University Medical Center opened their Cooperative Care Unit in April 1979. Their model includes an intensive educational experience for both the patient and a live-in family member or friend ("care partner"). They encourage full patient and family involvement in care, thereby preparing both parties for care at home after discharge. The planning process for this acute-care unit began fifteen years before. They included their trustees, administration, faculty, and staff as well as federal government health care authorities, Blue Cross–Blue Shield of Greater New York, and the New York State Department of Health (Grieco and others, 1990).

New England Deaconess Hospital of Boston, Massachusetts, is testing the benefits of patient empowerment in their eight-bed Cardiovascular Health Integrated (CHI) Unit (Pasternack, 1992). The CHI project task force developed a mission statement, action plans, and guidelines for the new model. The goals of the unit are to empower patients to participate in their own care decisions, to encourage patient and family involvement, to humanize and demystify health care, to maximize communication between professionals and patients, and to create an environment for healing. Care is personalized through encouraging patients to dress in street clothes, individualizing medication schedules, providing uninterrupted therapeutic sleep, having unlimited visiting hours, and encouraging family members to spend the night. Other components of the model include active patient and family participation, risk modification classes, and group patient/family education including stress management and training in eliciting the relaxation response.

Key success factors are the role of the primary nurse, who coordinates the care throughout the hospital stay, and multidisciplinary team rounds, which include the patient and family in developing the plan of care. The CHI Unit model will be studied and compared to the more traditional medically oriented model. Potential benefits that may be measured include:

A. Patient outcomes
    1. Increased patient/family satisfaction with care
    2. Improved self-efficacy scores

    3. Decreased need for emergent care for the year following discharge
    4. Earlier return to work
    5. Improved quality of life
    6. Fewer medical complications
    7. Increased knowledge
B. Staff outcomes
    1. Higher job satisfaction
    2. Decreased staff turnover
    3. Increased cooperation and collaboration among health care professionals
C. Institution outcomes
    1. Increased occupancy rates
    2. Decreased length of stay
    3. Improved utilization of hospital resources
    4. Other benefits derived from enhanced patient, nurse, and physician interaction and satisfaction

Most organizations find that patient and family empowerment is fully within the scope of their mission and values. As Scott exclaims, "What has taken us so long to realize that we are making a mistake? We must walk our talk." We must lift the veil and see our care from the patient's perspective and then be willing to make the changes. The following are strategies for empowering patients.

Counseling

Kaiser (1992) teaches that health care is ready for a new metaphor, that of a university. With this metaphor, disease or injury is viewed as an opportunity for learning about oneself and one's well-being. Nearly all who are ill or injured reflect on their lives, asking such questions as, "Why me?" "What has brought me to this?" "How did I become this ill?" People are often eager to explore the meaning of their lives and to look at how they are meeting their needs after the "wake-up call" of an illness or injury. It is an essential for patients to be facilitated by caregivers to use this natural time of reflection and exploration to promote an understanding of themselves, their needs, and their goals.

St. Charles helps caregivers work with patients in this way by offering a counseling series for staff members. This series involves discussion and practice of basic counseling skills such as active listening, positive regard, concreteness, confrontation, and information giving. The therapeutic relationship is taught as a process that begins with establishing the relationship, moves to facilitating exploration, and ends with developing a plan for action. Other topics include the nature of crisis, skills to elicit the relaxation response, and the "hardiness" factors: control, commitment, and challenge.

Patient and Family Education

When the metaphor for hospitals was the auto-repair shop, patient education was low on the priority list, often not thought of until the day before or the day of discharge. Now with shorter lengths of stay, more informed consumers, and research showing the value of patient education, health care needs to include patient and family education as an integral part of the whole process of care from preadmission to postdischarge. Implementation of patient and family education involves setting up the structure, gaining physician support, gaining staff commitment, providing the resources, and involving the family.

Setting Up the Structure. A key decision that has to be made when implementing patient education is who should be doing it. Many hospitals have created a position for a patient-education coordinator. This person usually creates the patient-education program, trains staff, and in some instances provides the education to patients. Although most hospitals make this a hospitalwide position, Planetree at California Pacific Medical Center in San Francisco, and at other locations, has made this a unit-based position. Haggard (1989) offers the following analysis of the benefits and drawbacks for hospitals trying to decide whether to create a patient-education coordinator or to keep the responsibility with the staff nurse.

Benefits	*Drawbacks*
Responsibility is with one easily identified person.	Nurses may abdicate their responsibility for teaching.
The coordinator can keep current with new information.	Teaching may not be done in coordinator's absence.
The coordinator can in-service all staff.	A hiring error will have a serious impact on the whole hospital.
Teaching tools can be screened and developed by the coordinator.	
Patient education can be evaluated in a consistent, organized way.	
An expert in patient education can be hired.*	

Other possibilities include the use of a hospitalwide education committee and the use of unit-based education committees. St. Charles uses a combination of all three approaches, including a quarter-time patient-education coordinator who also has some responsibility for community and medical education. The patient-education coordinator acts as a resource and central organizer for the committees. The hospitalwide committee decides on overall standards, resources, and approaches. The unit-based committees are a part of shared governance. Their role is to identify needs, to develop learning materials and approaches based on these needs, and to implement the recommendations of the hospitalwide committee. Each hospital must decide the best approach based on its unique resources and needs.

Gaining Physician Support. Regardless of the structure used, physician support and endorsement are essential. A 1983

---

*Adapted from *Handbook of Patient Education* by Ann Haggard, with permission of Aspen Publishing, Inc., ©1989.

American Hospital Association survey found that 42 percent of the hospitals questioned cited medical-staff attitudes as a hindrance to the development of patient-education programs (as cited by Haggard, 1989). The key to physician support is their involvement in information development. Physicians make a good point when they request that information provided by hospital staff be compatible with information provided by them. Nothing is more confusing to patients than to receive conflicting information. Even though physicians rarely have time to serve on education committees, it is important to offer them opportunities to review educational materials. The following are some strategies for obtaining physician support:

- Involve physician office staff in reviewing educational materials or as committee members.
- Send packets of information for physician review or input. Be sure to include a final date for return, with a notation that no response will be considered acceptance.
- Make it easy for physicians to initiate patient education.
- When presenting programs to the medical staff, be sure to have the product fully developed and complete. Haggard (1989) warns, "Never go to these meetings unprepared and ask the physicians to develop content. Not only will the process drag on forever but the doctors will not be able to agree, and the ensuing arguments may result in nothing being approved" (p. 11).
- Keep a high profile. Patient education should be at the forefront of hospital activities. Keep physicians informed of patient problems and progress. Be a true resource when patients need help. Monitor the value of patient education and make that value known.

Gaining Staff Commitment. Although educating patients has always been a key element of nursing practice, too often nurses work in a system that precludes their doing so effectively. The traditional system rarely includes a team approach, in which disciplines, including physicians, are all coordinated and centered on the patient and family. As a result, patient and family goals are not elicited, and there is a failure to develop an overall plan. This process leads to a "shift mentality," where staff members focus on patient needs only during their eight-hour shift and fail to develop long-range individualized goals such as preparation for discharge. Without support for continuity of care and time for patient education, staff members tend to focus on their tasks rather than on nursing process and patient and family learning.

With a patient-focused approach, patient and family learning becomes a central part of the team's efforts. Recommendations for implementation include the following:

- Include patient and family education as a part of both the team's and the hospital's mission and vision statements.
- Include patient and family learning needs and strategies as a part of the agenda for team meetings.
- Include teaching of patient-care plans. Include a review of learning needs and progress in the shift report.
- Integrate patient and family learning as targets in quality-assurance and patient-satisfaction surveys.
- Include patient and family education as a part of incentive and recognition programs.
- Perhaps most important, provide the time for patient and family education.
- Reorient the staff to coaching and facilitating rather than teaching. Every interaction with the patient and family can be used as an opportunity for learning.
- Remind staff of the importance of patient and family education through supervision and feedback.

Providing the Resources. Once staff members have the preparation and time, they need the tools. These tools include patient materials such as audiovisual materials, printed handouts, and computer programs, and staff tools such as standardized protocols and standards of care. St. Charles addresses this need for resources through its patient-education committee. The committee publishes a staff newsletter and develops instructional tools such as guidelines for patient education for various procedures and diseases, patient information fact sheets, and educational videotapes and audiotapes; it also runs staff seminars. Here is an example of some patient-education guidelines from a staff newsletter, excerpted from the *Patient Education Update* (Garnett, 1992, p. 3, courtesy of International Patient Education Council, Rockville, Md.):

- Adults learn best when there is a problem to be solved. Relate what the patient needs to know to what he perceives as the relevant problem or concern.
- Adults learn easiest when learning is connected to something familiar. Adults have a life time of experiences. Try to link the new to the old.
- Adults want to control their own learning. Let them state their goals. Consider pace and learners' confidence in their ability to learn.
- Adults need to be involved in the process. Establish the feeling that "we're in this together." Remember, doing is more effective than simply hearing or seeing.
- Adults need reinforcement of new information. To be effective rephrase the information and present it a different way.

Planetree has another approach. It offers a Health Resource Center, which provides a packet of information to patients who desire it. This information may be about any area of interest to patients as well as about their specific diagnosis and needs. This freestanding center is open to the community and offers medical and holistic health books as well as a list of agencies and a clipping file of current medical research.

Involving the Family. Probably the most significant determinant of success or failure in patient education is the patient's family, including friends who serve in a support role. Haggard (1989) emphasizes the importance of assessing how the family is coping before initiating teaching. Family members usually go through certain stages in their adjustment to their loved one's illness or injury similar to those encountered during grief. It is important to match interventions to the individual's needs during each stage. The following are the stages of adjustment:

1. Denial—shock and disbelief. This stage may be character-
    ized by rationalizing away symptoms and resisting treat-
    ment or clinging to unrealistic expectations.
2. Disorganization. Family members may be angry or may
    blame caregivers or each other.
3. Anxiety. This stage lasts until family members develop new
    ways to cope. They may be too overwhelmed to take in new
    information or make decisions.
4. Adjustment. Through support, time, and information, fam-
    ily members adjust to the patient's illness.

The most important intervention that caregivers can make
is to assist family members in their adjustment to the patient's
illness. The more support and help family members receive during early hospitalization, the more likely they will be able to
learn new information needed for home care. Also, when family members are kept well informed and feel like an important
part of the process, they are likely to trust the caregiver as a
source of information.

Nurturing, Supportive Environment

Patients and their families must feel that their caregivers care
about them personally, that they are present for them, and that
they are in control of their environment. Caregivers must assess patients' unique needs and ways of coping, then adjust approaches accordingly. For example, some patients do not want
information. A friend of mine recently told me about his hospital experience. "The last thing I wanted was information. My
nurse came and began teaching me about what to expect regarding my hip surgery. I felt more and more anxious. Finally I
told her, 'I don't want to know what's going to happen!'" Unfortunately, we sometimes forget the goal of all our efforts: to
meet the unique needs of each individual.

Active Patient and Family Participation

Generally the more patients and their families are informed
about and involved in their care, the better they do both in the

hospital and after they return home. Active participation is encouraged by having an open-chart policy, allowing medication self-administration, teaching self-care, and eliminating barriers to visitors. For example, patients on Planetree units are encouraged to read their charts, ask questions, or make their own notations. In response to common concerns of physicians and staff, Robin Orr, national director of hospital projects at Planetree (as cited by Kaiser, 1991c, p. 3), replies, "It doesn't make sense for people to be restricted from information about their condition. They deserve to read about planned treatments and current efforts to help them. Research has shown that litigation and malpractice come from mistrust. Planetree has created a trusting environment. We are silently telling the patients, 'We trust you.'"

Amenity Menus

These menus list a variety of enjoyable, educational, and transformational activities. Kaiser (1991b) suggests that amenity menus offer patients control over their care and access to various services and therapies. Many of the items can be provided by volunteers; others may have a surcharge. At St. Charles the teams plan to create menus for patients to choose from before they come to the hospital. These menus allow patients to decide, for example, whether to have their bath in the morning or evening, and they assess personal preferences for such things as back rubs, visiting hours, extent of family involvement in care, and relaxation training. Kaiser (1991b, p. 9) lists some possible amenities, including massage, visits from former patients who have recovered from a similar condition, visualization training, visit from a humorist, special meals and treats, life-skills training, and hydrotherapy.

Revised Outpatient Processes

Many hospitals have realized the futility of trying to complete admission procedures and at the same time teach outpatients about their condition on the morning of their surgery. St. Charles Medical Center created a preadmission process whereby patients are seen five to seven days before their admission. During this visit caregivers perform all tests and complete assessment and admission forms. They determine patient and family goals and begin to devise plans of care. Based on this assessment, they initiate education and offer an opportunity for relaxation training. This procedure has done much to empower patients and improve care. On the morning of admission caregivers welcome patients, answer any final questions, and escort the patient with family members directly to surgery.

Also, many times counseling to develop coping skills and to make life-style changes cannot be completed during the short span of a hospital stay. This is one reason why the shift to outpatient treatment at the end of a hospital stay is crucial. Not only can counseling and education started in the hospital be completed, but patients who are being case-managed in the community can receive education, support, and therapy. A good example of this kind of service is The Nursing Network and its Nursing Wellness Centers at Carondelet St. Mary's Hospital and Health Center in Tucson, Arizona (see Chapter Five).

Implementing Nontraditional Therapies

In Chapter Two we described several mind/body therapies: relaxation training, guided imagery and visualization, meditation, and counseling (including group therapy) as well as Therapeutic Touch and massage. Now we will explore how to implement these as well as other nontraditional methodologies in the hospital setting. First, we will explore the context for implementation as we look at the need for a customer-driven orientation and an organization that thrives on change. Then we will identify the desired leadership characteristics for introducing therapies that break from the established traditions. We close this section with a review of strategies for implementation and discuss common barriers and learnings.

Orientation to Customers

Leebov and Scott (1990) warn us, "We have tied ourselves unquestioningly to past practices, whether they still serve our interests or not. We have worshipped and glorified our traditions so much so that we now have trouble differentiating between those that work and those that do not. Change and experimentation are very sensitive, even political, issues because so many healthcare professionals interpret them as rejections of the hallowed traditions of the past" (p. 104). Yet, the times they are a-changing.

Perhaps health care needs to take a lesson from the auto industry. Many U.S. auto manufacturers failed to invest in research and development or new innovations. It took the near collapse of that industry to move them into change and CQI. Health care is on the verge of a similar crisis. Leebov informs managers that they have several options: "(1) You can watch what is happening. (2) You can make things happen. (3) You can wonder what happened. Option 2 is a necessity" (p. 107).

Pointing to a symptomatic problem, Lerner (1991) asks, "Why is it that Spiegel's research on the efficacy of group therapy for cancer patients goes largely ignored by the medical community? This research indicated that patients receiving group therapy had 2 times the survival time of those who did not receive group therapy. If this had been the effect of a drug, it would have made the headlines."

Health care as we know it is in danger of becoming a dinosaur. Medicine's myopic view of health, as well as its failure to accept credible research outside of its domain, puts it at risk of losing its credibility from the consumer's point of view. Sophisticated customers are expecting ever higher levels of quality and choice. Winston (1992) predicts that organizations that dominate during the 1990s not only will understand the changes that affect them but will use them to achieve ever higher levels of performance.

Leadership

Today's leaders must be eager, able, and willing to change. Winston calls for a new and daring leadership, "leadership that goes against the grain!" (p. 5). These are the kind of leaders who implement alternative therapies and other components of patient-focused healing. They share certain characteristics:

- They keep their eyes, ears, and minds open, searching for ways to improve on the system and enhance patient healing.
- They are willing to look at information from the patient's point of view.
- They are willing to take risks and the "heat" that goes with trying new things.
- They can rub the system the wrong way. "They challenge conventional wisdom, push the status quo, and attack 'sacred cows'" (p. 5).
- They develop programs from the customer's point of view.
- They are willing to begin wherever they can and with whatever they can. They do not get discouraged by not having money. They find ways to effect change anyway.
- They are willing to evaluate and improve their product on an ongoing basis.
- They are mavericks, people who ask provocative questions like, "Why do we do it this way?" and "What if?"

Winston (1992) considers these leaders heroes and describes six ways that they produce change.

1. They anticipate change. They realize they have a choice of whether to react defensively to change or to anticipate, promote, and lead change. They choose to move proactively.
2. They focus on high-leverage activities. They have little tolerance for bureaucracy. They work to overthrow systems and structures that hamper healing.
3. They select employees for their leadership qualities. Winston defines these as "the ability to see and articulate a clear compelling vision and mission, the will to see that the course is maintained, the courage to take a long-range perspective despite today's pressure, the willingness to empower others to remove impediments to success, the capability to display optimism, confidence, and courage" (p. 6).
4. They reward superior performance.
5. They prize courage and commitment. They lead by example, modeling integrity, results over busywork, innovation

over imitation, teamwork over personal gain, and risk-taking over conformity.

6. They communicate a clear and compelling vision. They exercise the courage of their conviction, focus on opportunities, and attract and energize people by offering an exciting and rewarding vision.

Nancy Petersen is one of these people. During a staff inservice, Nancy was listening to a young physician, David Redwine, present his innovative surgical technique for the treatment of endometriosis. Nancy listened carefully. Here were an entirely new method of diagnosing endometriosis and a treatment, using laproscopic surgery, that was highly successful. Nancy, recognizing that millions of women, five million in the United States alone, suffer with this disease and that little progress had been made in relieving their suffering, approached Dr. Redwine to learn more about his pioneering work. After reviewing the research, Nancy became convinced that the approach was a significant breakthrough. She pursued funding from the hospital to help Dr. Redwine with marketing and getting his treatment known and accepted by both consumers and the medical community. Then, she set out to let the world know. Working through the United States and Canadian Endometriosis Association and offering public lectures, she began spreading the word of hope for those suffering with endometriosis. Dr. Redwine continued to publish his work in professional journals and began speaking at national professional conferences. As more people became aware of his work, they came to St. Charles Medical Center in Bend, Oregon. As patients began coming to this rural part of central Oregon, they were often frightened by the remoteness. "Could the best treatment in the world really be found in this 180-bed hospital?" Nancy met with patients in their motel, in part because she anticipated their fear, but more to learn about their needs.

When I asked her what she attributed the success of her program to, she replied, "Dr. Redwine's treatment works. Many of the patients who come here have been to multiple physicians and have had multiple surgeries and drug trials. They often come in angry at the system. They have been ignored, placated, and told that their pain is all in their head. It takes a great deal of courage to come this far for a treatment when you have experienced so many failures. I also attribute our success to the fact that we listen to our patients, we care about them, and we follow through with what they tell us." Nancy shared two questions she always asks, "Are we meeting your needs?" and "How is your family or loved one doing with their stay here?" Nancy continued, "It's amazing how much patients will tell you if you ask. Our entire program is created around patient needs. If you listen, they will tell you what you need to know about their healing."

The Endometriosis Program at St. Charles now draws patients from Great Britain, Canada, Poland, Italy, and other countries. Some of these patients have returned to St. Charles for other surgeries as a result of their perception of the quality of care. Therefore, St. Charles is now a world-class health care facility. As this story shows, someone who shows initiative and vision can help increase a customer base for a hospital and contribute to patient healing.

Strategies

Nurses are likely to be the ones who implement complementary therapies such as Therapeutic Touch. Nurses do Therapeutic Touch because it helps their patients relax and helps relieve their pain. Yet, because it does not fit the traditional medical, biological model it is often scoffed at or ridiculed by physicians. One approach for introducing Therapeutic Touch is offered by this example from St. Charles.

After assessing the effectiveness of Therapeutic Touch with a number of patients and finding it to be a helpful tool in promoting relaxation and pain relief, I presented it to our surgeons. The first reaction was a resounding no! Clearly, as a group they felt this was an inappropriate modality for hospitalized patients. Later though, I had a number of physicians approach me and say, "Nancy, if this helps patients, I want you to know it is OK to do with my patients." As a result, I continued to offer Therapeutic Touch. Other nurses, having observed the positive benefits for their patients, asked to learn this approach. Now we have forty-five nurses who have received the training. Some of these nurses have gone to workshops outside of the hospital, and others have learned through workshops offered by the hospital. In addition, we have an ongoing group that meets on a weekly basis to practice, share learnings, and explore other methods of enhancing patient healing. In order to evaluate Therapeutic Touch, we have an ongoing program for questioning patients about their response. Because the responses have been overwhelmingly positive, we continue to offer this therapy.

This example describes an approach for implementing alternative treatments. Here are some other strategies. First, involve the board of directors early on and keep them informed of the rationale and progress. Second, do your research. Be prepared to justify the efficacy of your service. Kaiser advises, "The same evaluation criteria should be utilized for testing [an] alternative therapy, such as massage, as for evaluating any new drug or surgical procedure: Does it work? Under what conditions does it work? What are the contraindications? Is it worth the effort? (1991b, p. 2). As Borysenko (1991) points out, "What we do must be based in science. Science is the priesthood of our culture."

Third, be customer-driven. Solicit the customer's perspective. Customers include physicians and patients. Patients' views can be obtained through focus groups, surveys, and interviews. For physicians, a one-to-one interview is preferable. As Frances M. Buck of the Women's and Children's Center of the Community Medical Center in Missoula, Montana, relates about the creation of their program, "We met with thirty or forty physicians, at the very beginning, asking them for their thoughts, their involvement, and making them a part of the referral source as well as consultants to the program."

Fourth, make site visits to hospitals where alternative healing practices have been successfully implemented. These visits are an excellent resource because it is possible to see how the treatment works in practice. In addition, these visits build relationships with other hospitals with a like mission. Once these connections are established they become an ongoing source of information sharing, learning, and support. These visits also help sell your idea to others. Presenting a program that is successfully running is one of the best ways to convince nonbelievers.

Fifth, develop champions. Start with a few influential people before taking on the whole medical staff or the whole hospital. Not only does this strategy help develop supporters, but it also helps work out the flaws before going public. Scott, president of Mid-Columbia Medical Center, used both site visits and developing champions to sell his idea. "I didn't go before the medical staff as a group at first. It is too easy for a few people with strong opinions to dominate the group before you get a chance to inform them. Instead, we chose ten of our best physicians and fully informed them. Planetree consultants came to teach the Planetree concept; then we explored the question, 'Are we capable of doing this here?' We also had them talk with the board. We combined this approach with taking several key people, including physicians, their wives, and board members, to Planetree in San Francisco. Again, we asked the question, 'Aren't we capable of doing this?'"

Sixth, begin small. Kaiser (1991e) reminds us that it is difficult to change an entire organization. He recommends beginning by demonstrating the value of healing therapies on a special patient-care unit as a pilot project. "You need a 'safe harbor' for experimentation, training and data collection. You might call this unit a 'life-skills unit' or an 'integrated medical care unit.' Be certain that everyone on the unit (including doctors) supports what you are trying to do. Physicians and nurses not yet ready for this kind of thing can work on the other hospital units" (mesage 44).

Seventh, use volunteers whenever possible. There are many reasons for using volunteers. The most obvious is that they are cost-effective. This is a highly significant advantage in this time of shrinking reimbursement and shortages of professional staff. There are many other advantages, equally important. For example, there are talented people in our communities who would like to become involved in helping others. Peggy Carey, coordinator of oncology services at St. Charles, discovered many gifted people who were eager to donate their time in creating and facilitating support groups for cancer patients and their families. These people included a private therapist, community leaders (such as the director of the county mental health clinic), and hospital employees who wanted to volunteer in the community.

St. Charles also uses volunteers in a variety of other healing activities. Art in the Hospital is a volunteer service created and implemented by a local artist, Marlene Alexander. She organizes regular shows of local artists, advises the hospital in the purchase of art, and facilitates a support group for cancer patients and their families that uses art as a means of expression. Performance in the Hospital is a volunteer service created, facilitated, and supported by a local volunteer group, the United Compassionate Artists, with the help of Sarah Mason, RN. This group's mission is to bring healing to their community through the performing arts. They perform weekly at the hospital for both patients and staff. Their performances include music, poetry, and storytelling.

Sandy Mckinley started a "Mime Ministry" through the hospital's Pastoral Care Department after witnessing a tragic accident. She knew she wanted to bring solace and support to people suffering from illness and trauma. This sensitive and caring service has brought much healing and solace to patients and their families. Mckinley and Patty Riley, an enterostomal therapist, instituted a hospitalwide humor program in 1991. The program includes providing a humor cart for staff and patients as well as educational and awareness programs on the use of therapeutic humor. The humor cart contains toys, books, stuffed animals, and entertaining videotapes and audiotapes. The employee humor cart has been used to reduce stress in staff meetings. It helps by bringing a little levity to the staff's serious work.

Volunteers can also connect the hospital with important community organizations and services. Joan Klagsbrun and Constance Lorman of the Wellspring Center for Life Enhancement (Lexington, Massachusetts) developed a training program that prepares members of religious communities to visit with the seriously ill. The goal of the training is to form an ongoing support group that will continue to meet over time and work to-gether in a mutually supportive and empowering way to serve the needs of the seriously ill and disabled members of the community.

Mid-Columbia (as cited by Kaiser, 1991c) has become a model for the use of volunteers in community service. Their volunteer services include complementary facials and make-up applications, a "grandma" who rocks and cuddles sick children any time of the day or night, discharge partners who escort older patients home and help with a variety of tasks, and free transportation for seniors to medically related destinations.

Washoe Medical Center uses volunteers as patient repre-sentatives in their emergency room. Berkley Curtis (as cited by Kaiser, 1991c, p. 7) describes his work: "As a patient represen-tative, I work with the staff to support and empower patients and make their stay as pleasant as possible. . . . Being with the patient or family during a time of crisis, trauma or death, and knowing they are not alone, means so much to them. . . . Just knowing I might relieve someone's pain is enough reason to get up and celebrate." Much of the implementation and provision of patient-focused healing can be done by volunteers who heal themselves as they serve in healing others.

Eighth, develop a vision compelling enough and strong enough to move people forward during the turbulence of change. This is a key component. Yavapai Regional Medical Center (YRMC), Prescott, Arizona, received one of the two 1991 "21st Century Innovators" awards cosponsored by the Healthcare Fo-rum and 3M Health Care. The award was given on the basis of the vision of Pat Linton, former CEO; his vision is to transform YRMC into a total healing environment: "an environment where-in the people of YRMC work in partnership with patients and their families seeking peace of mind and peace of heart as well as physical cures or comfort because we understand the indivisible re-lationship that exists between body, mind, and human spirit" (Yavapai Regional Medical Center, 1991). Although Linton de-veloped the framework for the vision, he believes the people of YRMC will make it a reality. He has made it clear that every per-son has a role to play in this effort. Once the vision is created, it is imperative to communicate it clearly, succinctly, and continuously. Linton makes presentations to employees, the governing board, and the medical-staff executive committee. Also, steering committees address strategic areas of the plan, and a monthly newsletter informs and communicates about progress.

St. Charles used a slightly different strategy. During 1991 Lussier, the CEO, made healing health care a major goal of the organization. He designated a half-time director for the project and provided a budget for its definition and development. During the year the project was more clearly defined, brought into line with the hospital's mission, and communicated throughout the organization. He then began a vision-development process, which involved all members of the organization: the governing board, management, physicians, and staff. He used an outside facilitator to guide the process.

Ninth, build a supporting structure around the vision. One of the reasons healing programs fail is because they lack a context. Although the vision is the beginning of this context, more is needed. The CEO and top management staff must support the vision by being willing to expend money, time, and energy. Another important component of creating a context is forming a steering committee to guide and inform the process. The steering committee needs to include a cross-section of individuals critical to the program's success — for example, the vice-president for development, the CEO, the vice-president for personnel, physicians, a board member. In addition, subcommittees can deal with key areas such as culture development, organizational development, education, and communication.

Barriers and Learnings

Kaiser (1991e, message 276) asks, "We have a developed state-of-the-art. Why don't we use it?" The following are some of the barriers he has observed in organizations that fail in implementing innovative services.

- The overall vision and direction have not been well formed or clearly articulated, so no one has an overall view of where the organization is going.

- Too few people are involved in implementation.
- Strong political opposition forms internally.
- Top management is not sufficiently committed.
- Timing is not favorable.
- Appropriate rewards and punishments are not incorporated in the design.
- Values are contrary to personal or professional values.
- The effort is sabotaged by an outside group.
- The organization lacks maturity, energy, and stability.
- The effort is understaffed and underfunded.
- Mid-course corrections are not made.
- The implementation team lacks experience and training.
- The effort is overly dependent on outside resources.
- No one is assigned overall responsibility for the success of the effort.
- Consensus on the details is not gained.
- The implementation team is not powerful enough to overcome organizational resistance.

Kaiser offers here a valuable guide in undertaking new designs for organizations. The key to success is being open to learning both from our own mistakes and from those made by others.

In my experience at St. Charles, as director of the Healing Healthcare Project, I have my own lessons to share. I have a particular passion for implementing mind/body therapies. My initial direction with the project was to implement services such as therapeutic touch, counseling, Art in the Hospital, and Performance in the Hospital. I learned that some physicians and employees saw these services as "fluff." Their view was that if we want to affect patient healing, we need to address core issues such as inadequate staffing, noise, inconsistent assignments, and, fundamental to patient and family well-being, the cost of health care. As a result, we are focusing our attention also on healing the fundamental structure and processes for delivering care. Many of these changes are described in Chapter Four.

New Metaphors for Health Care

Kaiser encourages his readers to be conscious of the metaphors they use to think about their work. The most prevalent metaphor in health care is one of an auto-repair shop, where people are admitted, their bodies are repaired, and they leave. In this metaphor, health care providers are mechanics, and the patient's body is the vehicle. Kaiser (1991e, message 45) asks, "What would happen if we used different metaphors such as health care facility as theme park, or school, or cathedral? The answer is, we would change a lot of things as a result of the changed metaphors. The theme park focuses on the patient's experience. The school metaphor concerns itself with the patient's learning. The cathedral metaphor addresses the spiritual dimension of patients." All of these metaphors are needed. The future is about learning to manage multiple metaphors in our health care facilities.

Much of the work of healing in hospitals is about changing metaphors, about changing mind-sets. As we have shown, this is no small task. Implementing a healing environment changes the fabric and culture of the organization; it necessitates exploring and developing the hospital's mythology and vision. Also, it involves healing the care providers as well as the patients. Healing health care requires courageous leadership. It requires people who are willing to go against the grain in order to achieve a vision for health care and the people it serves. This vision is of health care that heals as well as cures. In the next chapter we will peer into this vision for the future.

Chapter 8

Envisioning
the Future

All things are ready if our minds be so.
William Shakespeare,
Henry V, act 4, scene 3

Needless to say the future of health care is blessed with uncertainty. In this chapter we will peer into the future as we intentionally design a "new civilization" for health care. This new era includes a full understanding and utilization of general systems theory, which broadens health care's focus from the person to the community and the environment. Also, grounded in the roots of a new learning society, health care takes a leadership role and collaborates with the government, the community, and the business sector to provide health education, resources, and care. There are care and compassion for all with an emphasis on medicine that incorporates high-tech, alternative, and complementary methods. Incentives for this model are both financial and altruistic, with an emphasis on personal accountability, volunteerism, and self-help approaches. After we review health care's present state, we will explore each of these aspects.

In order to shed some light on the future of health care in this country, the Healthcare Forum Leadership Center queried over 2,500 health care opinion leaders (400 responded). In addition, they conducted a series of focus groups, interviewed management experts, and reviewed the literature. They uncovered the following facts and perceptions (as cited by Curtin, 1992):

- Health care costs were almost 13 percent of the gross national product (GNP) ($738 billion) in 1991.
- In a Harris poll, 90 percent of Americans surveyed said there was need for a fundamental restructuring of the American health care system.
- Thirty-five million Americans lack health coverage; 75 percent of them are working citizens and their children.
- The cost for employee health insurance continues to rise at about 12 percent per year, absorbing nearly 50 percent of corporate profits. This cost is forcing some small businesses to drop health insurance benefits.
- Sadly, even in the face of this astronomical cost, our health outcomes, such as average life expectancy, morbidity, and infant mortality, are poor compared with those in other postindustrial societies.

Curtin identifies five megatrends that will mold these facts into new statistics:

1. An increase in highly invasive and expensive procedures, which funnel resources to the few.
2. Rising payer participation in determining resource allocation.
3. The failure of competition as a health care strategy. Competition has led to a fantastic waste of resources, contributing to less access and lower quality services.
4. An aging society with chronic, life-style-related diseases. "By 2015 we will have almost 60 million people over the age of 65 and 16 million over the age of 85" (p. 7).
5. A cost for maintaining the present system of $2 trillion per year, 17 percent of the GNP by the year 2000, with fewer and fewer people able to afford access to it.

Using these facts, perceptions, and statistics as a base, Forum presented their study participants with three possible futures:

1. Continued growth/high tech: Health care reform does not happen. High-tech advances continue extending lives and

providing cures but at high costs. The U.S. system continues to expand, reaching 17 percent of the GNP by 2001. Unequal access and medical indigency continue to increase. Patchwork coverage persists as managed care continues to expand.

2.   Hard times/government leadership: Universal access is mandated as a result of a persistent recession and political necessity. Health care costs decrease to 11 percent of the GNP by 2001, as a result of a frugal, Canadian-like system with significant rationing based on cost/benefit and outcomes research. Innovation decreases and heroic lifesaving advances decline.

3.   "New civilization": Health care changes on the basis of dramatic changes in science, technology, and society. Health care broadens its focus to include the community and environment. Managed care is accomplished through a government/business-sector partnership with discretion at the community level, as favored by national health-reform plans. This partnership provides a continuum of care, including health promotion and social health maintenance organizations, which are focused on supporting community health. Basic coverage is provided for all for both high-tech and alternative therapies and health care consumes 12 percent of the GNP in 2001.

Healthcare Forum found that nearly nine out of ten opinion leaders preferred the "new civilization" for health care. Yet, they thought it was the least likely to occur. They thought, by a slight margin, that the second possibility was the most likely of the three to become reality. Curtin admonishes us, "The only reason to predict the future is to prepare for its coming or to change its direction or pace. . . . In the end, the future will become what the present people want. Really want. Want badly enough to change their minds and habits for. Want badly enough to work and save for. Want badly enough to pay the price for" (p. 8).

The New Civilization

The year is 2000. Sarah Evans and her husband have just found out Sarah is pregnant with their first baby. But that's not all they found out. Their home computer, with its bioelectromagnetic analyzer, not only tells them of Sarah's pregnancy, it also reports the genetic makeup of the baby and outlines a plan for maximizing the health of each family member. When Sarah and David first married, they merged their health information into one system. Even before the pregnancy, they knew the likely genetic blueprint of their baby.

The early models for this type of information technology were available in the early 1990s. Vergil Slee, promoter of the Problem-Knowledge Coupler System, recognized the value of the program. This guidance system, created by Lawrence Weed, was a set of medical problem-solving and decision-support software. The function of the program was to keep the information in the patient's medical record organized around each of the patient's problems and to use the computer to couple (compare) each of the patient's problem-specific profiles with the literature (knowledge) about that problem and its management. According to Slee, "By creating a direct shortcut from the patient's problem to the knowledge about the problem in medical literature, Weed has provided a powerful guidance tool for the physician and the patient" (phone conversation, 1993). These files contained all the patient attributes (genetic, historical, and social) as well as symptoms, signs, and results of laboratory work. The computer was well suited to cope with the information-handling difficulties generated by the rate medical knowledge was accumulating, which was faster than a human being could read.

Sarah and David review their holistic plan of care, which outlines recommendations for the care of the whole person: mental, physical, emotional, and spiritual. Under mental recommendations, Sarah and David have access to the latest information on pregnancy and parenting, including a list of local classes and resources. The physical component outlines exercise, dietary, and monitoring (weight, blood pressure) recommendations, including parameters for the items Sarah is to monitor. If necessary, these parameters will alert her to seek consultation. Based on her health profile, the program recommends a nurse-midwife for her delivery. After reviewing the genetic profile, Sarah and David learn that the baby has a 10 percent chance of developing cancer in her lifetime. Recommendations are outlined to reduce the risk, taking into account the fact that genetic makeup is constantly being altered by environmental factors such as stress, life-style, chemicals, and toxins, as well as random mutations. They learn that the cancer risk can be reduced to 5 percent by following dietary recommendations early in the baby's life.

The emotional and spiritual recommendations are tailored to their needs and values. Sarah loves her work, and David wants to be a dad more than anything on earth. The program reminds them of their values, recommends natural-childbirth classes so they both can participate in the birthing process, and suggests a regular schedule of quiet time together where they focus on bringing peace and love to the new baby.

Sarah's sister, Ann, who has a number of physical problems, had a physician recommended for her care and delivery. The genetic profile for her baby indicates a high probability of diabetes. Ann and her physician are considering genetic engineering. Both Ann and her husband are receiving counseling for emotional support and treatment planning.

Harry Smith enters some disturbing symptoms he is having into his health program. After integrating his symptoms with information from his bioelectromagnetic analysis, the computer informs him he has gallstones. The computer suggests a number of treatment options, all with their risks and benefits. Harry chooses laproscopic gallbladder removal, one of the top two recommendations. Also, he chooses from a number of options for anesthesia, deciding not to use medications. Via the computer, he notifies his office that he will need to take two days off for the surgery, including recovery, and he schedules the mobile health van to arrive later that morning. Again using the computer, he sends the surgeon his health profile and treatment choices. When the van arrives, the surgeon and nurse perform the surgery. The surgery is painless as Harry wears virtual-reality (VR) goggles and listens to his favorite music throughout the process. The nurse stays with Harry for a few hours while he recovers. During this time she teaches him skills for speeding the healing process through guided imagery and relaxation, and supplies dietary, exercise, and other information for his care.

Sharon Nelson is the unfortunate victim of a severe auto accident: the results are loss of function in her right arm and paraplegia caused by spinal-cord damage. She is stabilized at her local hospital, then transferred to one of the high-tech centers located strategically throughout the nation. A team of multidisciplinary practitioners quickly assess her needs and develop a holistic plan of care. She is taken to surgery, where she will have micromachines (developed from nanotechnology) implanted to begin the process of nerve and muscle repair in her arm. Her injured spinal cord is injected with human nerve-growth factor.

A multiskilled, holistic practitioner works intensively with Sharon and her family. He takes time to assess their belief system and methods of coping, as well as information from bioelectromagnetic scanning. Sharon's bedside computer provides a plan of care for Sharon and her family to review and revise as they desire. Once completed, the plan is the blueprint for care. Nutritional therapy, including medicinal herbs, are intentionally prepared with healing prayer. Environmental sensors are synchronized to maximize the healing potential of the bioelectromagnetic field. Her family chooses to stay in the adjacent room so they can participate in her care. A therapeutic relationship is established, and every conversation and action is intentional in order to promote Sharon's healing. Sharon chooses from a list of alternatives for relaxation and pain control, ranging from acupuncture to VR to nonaddictive medications.

Wanda Scott, now eighty years old, is admitted to the hospital after a stroke. She also has degenerative arthritis and congestive heart failure. In the year 2000, she is not eligible for the high-tech treatment available to younger victims of heart disease and neurological disorders. And that is just fine with Wanda. At this point, she, like most of her peers, is more interested in the quality of her life than in the quantity. Wanda is admitted to the acute-care area of the healing village. The goal of her treatment is to stabilize her condition and to empower her by providing her with knowledge and methods to enhance her healing and quality of life.

Wanda feels better just from being in the healing village. The design is soft and nurturing. It feels like home, with lots of natural light and views of nature. She looks out on a beautiful garden, where she can see and hear the birds, waterfalls, and streams. The plants are all the colors of the rainbow. She feels energized by the view. Later she realizes that these are organically grown herbs, fruits, and vegetables, as well as flowers, which are used as medicinal and nutrient therapies.

She is cared for by a multiskilled, holistic practitioner. After an assessment of her needs, beliefs, and coping skills, a plan for her care is developed. Her caregiver finds that Wanda believes her life is coming to a close soon, and her main goal is to maintain as much independence as she can in the time she has left and to prepare herself emotionally and spiritually for life's end.

Wanda chooses not to use her bedside computer—she never did like the things—so her caregiver enters all the information from her assessment along with values and preferences. The computer provides treatment options with their risks and benefits. After reviewing them, Wanda creates her treatment plan. She chooses a combination of medications, physical therapy, acupuncture, life-span counseling, and spiritual healing. Her caregiver helps her create a treatment schedule. Because Wanda no longer has any family, she is connected to a local teenager, Sue. Sue is volunteering as a part of a class about altruism. Sue has been volunteering now for a full year and has decided to make this kind of service a regular practice. Sue explains, "It is so rewarding to help others. Being a volunteer has really helped me find out who I am and that I can make a difference in the world." After four days of intensive treatment Wanda is discharged from the acute area to the assisted-living center.

The assisted-living center carries on the plan of care; it emphasizes the active participation and involvement of its clients. Clients who are able care for children in on-grounds day-care centers and help tend the gardens, grounds, and animals of the healing village. Also, they may choose to act as healing volunteers themselves, assisting others in need. Wanda chooses to use the many skills she learned for her own healing in helping others. One of her clients, Elizabeth, is dying from a terminal illness. Wanda sits with Elizabeth daily, helping her review her rich life and discuss any unfinished business. Elizabeth particularly likes the therapeutic touch Wanda offers each afternoon before she leaves. Elizabeth comments, "It is so wonderful to have Wanda visit. We both have so much in common, and I know she is with me because she truly cares. I feel like I'm helping her too. That is an important part of my own healing."

The early models for these kinds of healing centers were created in the early 1990s. Earl Bakken, inventor of the first implantable pacemaker and a board member of North Hawaii Community Hospital, a fifty-bed hospital in Kamuela, Hawaii, spearheaded the creation of this new model for hospitals. According to Pat Linton, CEO, the initial planning, involving community members and an expert in psychoarchitecture, began in 1990 (Linton, 1991). Their vision for a healing village incorporated architectural and grounds design as well as therapeutic services and programs. They also planned to integrate many of the healing traditions of the rich, diverse cultures found on the island with allopathic medical treatments.

As Linton (1991) outlines the plans, they will use the grounds and architecture as instruments of healing by incorporating the healing powers of nature. For example, they will use as much natural light as possible, and water will be an integral part of the gardens. These gardens will truly be healing as they will include medicinal herbs and organic vegetables and fruits that can be used as nutrients and therapies. In addition, the planting design will use colors to affect chakras (energy centers of the human body) in ways conducive to healing. There will also be ohana, or family rooms, waiting and education areas, as well as areas for quiet meditation or consultation and examination and treatment rooms that can be used for allopathic, massage, or acupuncture treatments. All these areas will include music and will be nurturing, soft spaces where patients can have control over their environment.

In addition, the planners are exploring with complementary religious and ethnic groups the use of such methods as Buddhist meditation, Kahuna healing, prayer, and acupuncture. They plan to use cross-trained teams of caregivers who will use guided imagery, therapeutic touch, relaxation methods, and other therapies outlined by the American Holistic Nurses' Association, as well as traditional techniques. In addition, Linton envisions a department of healing services to promote mind/body/spirit healing. Staff members with skills in chaplaincy, nursing, and counseling will assist patients and family members in learning how to tap into their own healing potential. They will also support hospital staff in their healing and skill development.

Now we will look at three forces that will shape the new civilization of health care: general systems theory, the model of a learning society, and an advanced stage of medicine known as Era III medicine.

General Systems Theory

General systems theory offers a new paradigm not only for health care but for all society. "Society [has] become so complex that traditional ways and means are not sufficient anymore. Approaches of a holistic or systems nature have to be introduced" (Bertalanffy, 1983, p. 21). Kuhn (1970), who was responsible for equating the idea of a paradigm shift with scientific revolution, used the word *paradigm* to mean shared premises and values that determine the nature of scientific inquiry. The dominant paradigm of a society is influential because it determines the kinds of questions scientists and others in that society are prompted to ask.

The mechanistic approach to science fixed certain attitudes and ways of viewing the world, encouraging health care providers to view patients as cases or body parts and employers to view workers as units or equivalents. The mechanistic model of science has its place and has contributed many major achievements in health care, such as those in biomedical research and genetics. Yet the mechanistic model has failed to explain many aspects of life. For example, the mystery of embryonic development defies mechanistic science, and the biological phenomenon of equifinality is another major embarrassment to mechanistic theory. Equifinality is the organism's inner-directed ability to protect or restore its wholeness. In biology the most dramatic form of equifinality is regeneration, as when a lizard grows a new tail.

Bertalanffy used the concept of equifinality as proof that organisms are goal-seeking, that they behave purposefully to maintain their condition or achieve their intended condition (Davidson, 1983). He linked biology with teleology to suggest that an ultimate purpose is apparent in nature. As we suggested earlier in this book, a sense of purpose and of having choice and control in one's life significantly influences health. Yet medical science, with its root in mechanistic science, excludes such "soft" variables because they are not quantifiable. When integrating healing and curing into health care, a paradigm is required that is large enough to include "soft" variables such as ultimate purpose as well as more easily quantifiable variables. General systems theory offers such a paradigm.

Now we will expand our definition of systems thinking, which we began in Chapter Four. Here are some of its key tenets, which we will draw on later as we outline the map for a new civilization in health care.

A system is composed of smaller systems and is also a part of larger systems. For example, within a person are many systems interacting with one another. This is evident on an intracellular level and intercellular level, on an organ and an organ-systems level. At the same time, the wholeness of the person interacts with the environment. This same process occurs on an interpersonal level, a community/societal level, a national/international level, a planetary/stellar level, and a galactic/universal level. These systems are organized in a hierarchical pattern of ascending levels of organized complexity.

The common denominator of these systems within systems is interaction. *A system is a whole that functions as a whole as a result of the interaction of its parts.* Another key characteristic of systems is a manifestation of something intangible yet quite real, its organization. *A system has a pattern, a form that is unique to that system.*

Human beings are more than their constituent ingredients of water and other substances such as protein, carbon, fat, minerals. They are the organization of their parts. Disrupt that organization, and they die. To look at it another way, although the cell population of the human body repeatedly dies and is replaced, people survive because their organization survives. Human life is an expression of a universal force of organization, a force that coordinates about 10 billion cells in the brain and approximately 100 trillion cells in each body. "It is a force like gravity, that is too mysterious to explain—nobody knows what gravity is—but it is too common to ignore" (Davidson, 1983, p. 26).

A system is greater than the sum of its parts because the system consists of the parts plus the way the parts interact and relate to each other and the qualities that emerge from that relationship. Herein lie the limitations of the mechanistic, analytic approach to science and medicine. In dissecting and studying the parts we know only the parts. We do not know the whole. The components of a system display the full range of their true nature only through their interaction among themselves and with their environment. For example, an individual will act differently when part of a group of friends than when he or she is part of a group of strangers.

Systems thinking is vital to our understanding of health; yet we tend to focus on health problems in isolation. We fail to include the problems' contexts. As a result, we often fail to solve our most vexing problems. For example, the search for a cure for cancer has to be linked through a whole continuum of systems from the gene to the solar system, as evidenced by the effects of the sun on the development of skin cancers.

The scope of the search for a cure for cancer suggests another important concept in systems thinking: *boundary definition.* In the attempt to resolve a problem, boundary definition, what is included in the perspective, must be wide enough to include all the relevant factors. With general systems thinking one must be continually aware of suboptimization, or failure to examine a sufficiently broad picture. Kaiser (1991e, message 52) challenges health care: "It is time to think about a hospital without walls. We first thought of the hospital as a place. Then, we began to think about it as a system. It is now time to think about the hospital in terms of the area it serves."

Kaiser advises hospitals to draw a ring around their institution. Although hospitals can make this ring as large as they like, they must realize they are accountable for the health of everyone within its boundary. Imagine hospitals being truly accountable for the health of the people they serve, truly being "health care." Viewed from a systems perspective, hospitals are as accountable for the people outside their walls as they are for those within them. To care for the health of people includes much more than tending them when they become sick. To care for the health of people means paying attention to their education, their environment, their social support systems, their work life, and their home life. Viewed from a systems point of view, the health care system interacts with the school system, the mental health system, the social welfare system, the criminal justice system, business and industry, churches, the public health system. No one system can do it alone. All are in a process of mutual interaction. The question is how to have these multiple systems blend to improve the health status of the population they jointly serve. When we view health care in this way, we can see that collaboration, cooperation, pooling of resources, and networking are all vital.

Systems thinking is the foundation of TQM because TQM should apply not only to what goes on within an organization but also to what happens or does not happen outside the organization. One Utah hospital provides a model of this view. The challenge the hospital was facing was how to provide medical care for the increasing numbers of critically ill newborns. The first inclination was to recruit a neonatologist. But instead the hospital did a remarkable thing — it looked outside its walls and examined the care of the pregnant mothers before they came to the hospital. It found that a number of them were poor and had failed to obtain prenatal care. As a result, the hospital started a prenatal clinic for low-income mothers. Its efforts have resulted in a decrease in the numbers of premature births. Caregivers there are now seeing healthier babies.

When we view human beings as systems within systems, the need becomes obvious for a holistic approach to care and medicine. Also, it becomes clear that we need to look beyond the body in order to understand and treat illness. A "cure" for any condition may be of little help if the patient returns to an "ill" environment. Many times the best procedure, medication, or treatment has been negated by environmental factors. One example is the patient who has cardiac bypass surgery for heart disease yet continues to smoke, eats a high-cholesterol diet, and returns to a high-stress environment.

With systems thinking we at last have a paradigm fitting for twenty-first-century health care. Yet even this paradigm has its limitations. We need a science of life that encompasses all its features. This science will accommodate such intangibles as consciousness, paranormal phenomena, bioelectromagnetics, and acupuncture. For example, some evidence from bioelec- tromagnetics suggests that "living processes may in fact be fun- damentally electromagnetic in nature, since novel evidence sug- gests that life forms emit extremely low level electromagnetic [EM] radiation. Thus, EM fields may be formative to life rather than explicable in terms of what is already known, thwarting any possible explanation in terms of conventional science" (Rubik, 1992, p. 21). Perhaps, herein lies a question about the future of hospitals and physicians, the present primary sources of health care. Is health care only about the treatment of disease and in- jury or is it about life?

Toward a Learning Society

In this section we present the case for a learning society as the model for the new civilization. Harman and Hormann (1990) remind us that the desire to create is a basic urge. "Fundamen- tally, we work to create, and only incidentally do we work to eat. . . . One of the great disservices of the modern paradigm is that it obscured the fact of our creative urge, and persuaded us that we really are economically motivated and work for economic reward" (p. 26). The overriding focus on mere economic growth and technological advance, unguided by overarching values, is becoming increasingly intolerable. The need is for a new, more sustainable and enriching focus. For example, the present production economy can no longer provide challenging work. Also, because of the many technological successes of our time, all the labor force is no longer needed. The solution has been to create the perception of increased need. Yet we are finding that limitless consumption of materials and services eventually runs into difficulty. We live in a finite universe, and our planet's resources are limited. However, although full employment is no longer needed, full participation is essential from a social standpoint. People basically seek meaningful activities and relationships. They thrive on challenge.

So what is the answer, given that the production economy will eventually fail to provide enough work roles? Harman and Hormann (1990) offer two possibilities: The first is continuation of the transfer-of-income payments from some source such as governments, institutions, or individuals to people deemed needy or worthy. This approach has not proven fruitful in the past. The second possibility is to move toward a learning society. This approach involves a more fundamental transformation of society than transfer-of-income payments. It is feasible because it answers the question raised earlier: "When it no longer makes sense for an economically and technologically successful society to have economic production (and consumption) as its central focus, what then becomes that society's 'central project'?" According to Harman and Hormann (1990) there is only one satisfactory answer: "Learning and human development, in the broadest possible sense — as an end as well as a means. Learning about self, health, meaning in life; learning skills to be used in service or productive creation; learning that the potentialities for learning are endless" (p. 31). The blueprint for health care's future is revealed.

Health care is at a pivotal juncture. If it chooses a healing paradigm and defines its mission as life, health, and wellness as well as the treatment of disease, it has to take a leadership role in the transformation of society to a learning society.

Much of the groundwork is laid. It need only be accepted and brought into the mainstream of health care and medicine. One need look only to the holistic health movement, which is based on the following principles. The first is that illness is opportunity, illness is a part of life. Illness need not be seen as the enemy or as the failure of a process of living. Evidence lies in the very nature of the immune system's development. It is through exposure to certain diseases such as cold viruses that the immune system matures. Also, our inability to hide from disease is surely an indicator that in some way disease is a part of living; we cannot have one without the other, just as we cannot appreciate beauty without ugliness or darkness without light. Not only does illness or injury help us appreciate and recognize health, it also offers an opportunity to learn — to learn about oneself and one's needs, as well as about attitudes, habits, or beliefs that may need changing.

Clearly, illness, injury, and disease are part of humanity's living feedback system, telling us when we are off course. Consider your last cold. Was it an undeniable reminder that your body and soul needed rest? Consider, too, on a larger scale, the role of disease in overpopulation and as a reminder to the human consciousness of its responsibility for the health of its home, the earth, the universe. Poignantly, we look at our struggle to eliminate cancer, now recognizing the many environmental factors involved. In a sense, disease is an indicator that tells us the extent to which we have ruined our environment. For example, consider the link between skin cancer and the thinning of the ozone layer of our atmosphere and the multiple cancers resulting from exposure to chemical and radiation pollution.

The holistic health movement has as a second principle an open definition of health. Health is defined in much broader ways than simply as the absence of disease. Health and wellness imply being integrated, being whole in body, mind, and spirit; feeling energized with a sense of well-being; living up to one's potential and feeling aligned with one's purpose in life, all enhanced by an attitude of accountability and continuous learning.

The third principle is the need to practice preventive medicine. Disease prevention includes continuous learning through public education and followthrough with immunization, as well as sanitation.

The fourth principle posits the presence of an inner healer — the belief that a person knows naturally how to develop, heal, and prevent diseases. An inner healer is available for "consultation" — advice on treatment and prevention. This is a metaphor for taking the time to check in with one's own inner wisdom, to relax and focus inward on the subtle messages and wisdom of the self. Learning from one's self also supports people's religious and spiritual sense because their personal belief system is part and parcel of this inner wisdom.

The fifth principle is that the person is an integrated, interactive system involving the environment, body, mind, and spirit. This is not a new view of life. It is fundamental in Native American traditions. Native Americans have long recognized the inexorable unity of body, mind, and spirit with the environment of the earth and the "creator." With this view, people will continually learn from their environment and from themselves.

The sixth principle is that people should be responsible and accountable for their health instead of relying on a physician to "fix" them. More and more we are now documenting with research the power of self-help when people are provided with information and support. Likewise, we are documenting the dangers of dependence and the futility of trying to "fix" those who do not take an active role in maintaining their own health.

The seventh principle is that there is value in group help, which has proven to be an effective method for healing and learning about self. Alcoholics Anonymous, a pioneer of the group-help movement, has been so effective it has become a social movement in its own right. The Alcoholics Anonymous approach serves as a model for self-help groups of all varieties and types. This model utilizes a spiritual approach in the "twelve steps" program. These steps include admitting powerlessness over the use of alcohol, recognizing the need for help from "a power greater than myself," taking moral inventory, admitting problems to others, trying to make amends to those persons harmed in the past, seeking contact with God "as we understand him," and supporting others both socially and spiritually.

Finally, in the holistic health movement, alternative or complementary treatment methods are utilized out of a sincere desire to have patients participate in the reality of healing. These methods include acupuncture, acupressure, massage, imagery, and visualization. Congress is prodding the National Institutes of Health to support studies evaluating alternative therapeutic approaches. The newly created Office for the Study of Unconventional Medical Practices is charged with evaluating acupuncture, so-called folk remedies, use of herbs, homeopathy, naturopathy, nutritional treatments, massage therapy, and other therapies now outside of mainstream medical therapy in this country, although these therapies are not outside the mainstream in other countries. For example, Payer (1988) tells us that most practitioners of homeopathy in Europe receive an M.D. degree before they study homeopathy.

With a learning model as a foundation for society, we will turn now to the specifics of health care.

Era III Medicine

Dossey (1989), a physician of internal medicine with the Dallas Diagnostic Association, describes medicine as having certain periods or eras. Era I, "materialistic medicine," has existed for the past 100 years. Era I medicine focuses primarily on the material body. This view of health is based on the laws of energy and matter formulated by Isaac Newton some 300 years ago. This perspective views the universe and human beings as functioning along mechanistic lines. According to this view, all forms of therapy must be physical in nature, and the effects of the mind or consciousness are irrelevant. Era I brought tremendous advances in healing and our understanding of disease, including such advances as understanding the mechanisms of infection. As a result, antibiotics were developed, and people no longer risked death from simple pneumonia or risked losing a limb from a simple wound.

In the 1970s Era II, or mind/body, medicine began to

emerge. With Era II, a link was recognized between the mind or consciousness of a person and the physical state of the body. Medicine was able to show scientifically that emotions, attitude, and beliefs affected the body. "All the major diseases of our day—heart disease, cancer, hypertension, and more—were shown to be influenced, at least to some degree, by the mind" (p. 264). As a result of Era II medicine, a variety of therapies, such as biofeedback, relaxation therapy, and meditation, have been offered along with Era I approaches. The fusing of Era I and Era II medicine led to the entirely new field of medicine called psychoneuroimmunology.

Dossey envisions an advanced stage of medicine that is only now beginning to emerge in Western medicine—Era III, or "nonlocal medicine." Although Era III medicine recognizes the causal power of consciousness, it does not see this consciousness as limited to the confines of the individual human body or the single lifetime of a person. "Rather, in the Era III view, minds are spread through space and time; are omnipresent, infinite, and immortal; and are ultimately one. . . . Unlike Eras I and II, in Era III health and healing are not just a personal but a collective affair" (p. 265).

Because of this nonlocal view of the mind, Era III medicine constitutes a fundamental shift. *Nonlocal* is a term borrowed from quantum physics; it describes the ability of elementary particles to influence one another through distant space. This view of medicine is supported by the "prayer study" of cardiologist Randolph Byrd. Byrd (as cited by Dossey, 1989) conducted a ten-month study of 393 coronary patients at San Francisco General Hospital. Patients were assigned either to a group that was prayed for by home prayer groups (192 patients) or to a group that was not prayed for (201 patients). The study was a randomized, prospective, double-blind experiment, meaning it used the most rigid criteria in clinical studies. The nurses and physicians did not know which groups the patients were in.

Byrd's findings were astounding. Those in the group that was prayed for were five times less likely to require antibiotics and three times less likely to have the complication of pulmonary edema (a condition in which fluid backs up into the lungs because the heart is not pumping effectively); none of the prayed-for group required ventilator support for respiration as compared with twelve in the group not prayed for. As Dossey exclaims, "If the technique being studied had been a new drug or a surgical procedure instead of prayer, it would almost certainly have been heralded as some sort of 'breakthrough'" (p. 46).

These findings sound very fantastic when we draw on the old paradigms of science for our understanding. Yet there are parallels in the new physics. John Wheeler, physicist and cosmologist, has proposed three eras for physics. Era I physics is represented by the work of Galileo and Kepler, and Era II by the insights of Einstein, Newton, and Faraday. According to Dossey, Wheeler describes Era III physics as "'meaning physics' . . . because when observers 'put to use' various measurements at the quantum level of nature, meaning arises" (p. 266).

Era III medicine recognizes and complements the achievements of Eras I and II medicine. Dossey warns that some people interpret the discovery of the therapeutic potential of the mind as meaning therapy must become "all mind." "But just as Era III physics did not eliminate or discard Era I and Era II physics, but subsumed them, so, too, does the Era III 'medicine of nonlocality' subsume those forms of therapy that went before it" (p. 267).

In fact, equally exciting advances are occurring in Era I medicine. Goldsmith (1992) informs us of powerful new tools produced through the biotechnology revolution. He foretells that genetic therapy and immunotherapy will enable us to prevent most illnesses altogether. These technological advances alone will force the reinvention of the health care system. "The advances of biotechnology will have dramatic impact on critical care, allowing the sickest patients to heal more rapidly and sharply reducing lengths of stay, [and] on the treatment of heretofore hopeless diseases such as Alzheimer's and Parkinson's" (p. 34).

Examples of these advances include bioengineered human-growth factors, such as epidermal growth factors; advances in immune suppression for organ transplant, which are anticipated to decrease lengths of stay by 60 to 70 percent; and improvements in the treatment of hospital-acquired infections, which promise sharp reductions in the death rate (now 60,000 to 100,000 patients per year) as well as reduced ICU stays and improved results for patients. Other exciting examples include advances in the treatment of cancer. According to Goldsmith, "Advances in understanding of the genetic and cellular origins of cancer, and parallel advances in drug design, have fundamentally changed this process. Researchers now look for the vulnerable sequence of molecular events in cancer, and try to intervene to alter the course of disease" (p. 36). In addition, ambulatory surgery is predicted to account for 85 percent of all surgery by the end of the 1990s as a result of technological advances such as laproscopic surgery and early intervention in chronic diseases such as diabetes. As a result of these advances Health Futures (as cited by Goldsmith, 1992) predicts managed care will increase by 50 percent, inpatient hospital use will continue to decline, as will length of stay for transplant surgery, surgical rates, and the cancer death rate.

The Role of Health Care in Era III

Now, what is the role of health care? Although Goldsmith (1992) limits hospitals to acute care when he says, "While hospitals can act as catalysts for system change, the ultimate control points for health services use will lie outside the hospital" (p. 40), we believe hospitals can choose to take an expanded role. Hospitals need not limit their mission to the walls of their institution. In reality, to do so is sheer folly from a systems point of view. Hospitals have a tremendous nucleus of professional expertise and talent. Using this talent in partnership with the community and working collaboratively with government programs make tremendous good sense in a learning society.

As the reader may recall, almost 90 percent of the participants in Healthcare Forum's research preferred the "new civilization," where managed care is accomplished through a government/business-sector partnership with discretion at the community level. In this section, we will paint a picture of the new civilization in health care, which we shall call Era III health care.

Era III health care is a collaborative partnership of providers, businesses, citizens, government agencies, and government assistive plans focused on healing in their geographic area. These entities pool portions of their financial resources to further the purpose of health care. In addition, citizens and businesses volunteer time and contribute services to assist in enhancing their community's healing. Volunteerism is the norm, based on both its potential for enhancing self-healing through the beneficial effects of altruism and an understanding that the healing of any one member of society is related to the health of the whole. With the shortened workweek of the learning society, more people are unemployed and more time is available for altruistic activities.

With Era III health care, managed care is truly future-oriented. At birth, people receive their genetic assays and health care plans. Each plan identifies risk factors and recommends interventions to reduce these risks. Individuals with high risks or with poor support systems are linked with care coordinators, who are skilled in high-touch therapies such as counseling to help these families or individuals stay on track with plans of care.

Helping people in this way is part of the ethics of this more evolved form of health care. Ethics holds a central focus in Era III. Friedman (1991) articulates the key tenets: that "Protecting patients is the healthcare professional's highest calling. Providers have, first and foremost, two ethical responsibilities. One is to ensure that all people regardless of income or race or diagnosis, have access to necessary healthcare on a timely basis. The other is to ensure that patients receive the best care possible" (p. 14). Within this framework people are treated with dignity and respect as unique individuals possessing physical, emotional, intellectual, social, and spiritual needs. These are the primary ethical responsibilities of Era III caregivers, not making scientific or technological breakthroughs or protecting professional standing. Within this framework, health care is focused more on exploring questions than it is on providing answers. Within this framework also, each new advancement in science is expected to enhance the integrity of the human spirit and the environment. We owe this expectation to our patients, to ourselves, to the society that invests its trust in us.

Now that the economic incentives lie in enhancing health and reducing the utilization of event-driven medicine, hospitalization, and social programs, community programs are focused on child, family, and work-life health. Centralized social wellness and health centers, which are linked with hospitals, schools, churches, and businesses, are located in every community. These centers provide an entire continuum of care, including health education and prevention; treatment by nurse practitioners; alternative therapies such as naturopathy, acupuncture, massage, herbal therapies; counseling and mind/body/spirit therapies; allopathic medical care; mental health services; child and family services; criminal justice services; and environmental services.

As the hub of the health care system, these centers act as integrators and coordinators. People who are at risk, as indicated by genetic assay or lack of psychological or social support, are referred to the center at birth. The care of these at-risk people is coordinated by multiskilled professionals, who maintain regular contact and act as resources, educators, and mentors. The professionals see only the families most in need of their expertise and make referrals to other services as needed. After an initial assessment most families are followed by volunteer mentors and support people. These volunteers receive special education in parenting skills, therapeutic presence, counseling skills, and basic assessment skills. They stay connected with the center through regular support meetings and interactive computers. They are constantly updated on resource options and new methods for supporting and helping others. Also, the community health centers offer programs and courses on human potential, financial health, and conscious living and conscious dying. Individuals and families use the center as a primary health resource and may choose to be linked to the center through interactive computer networks.

As the central integrator of health, the center uses computer networks to identify best treatment approaches for illness and injury, environmental risks, and social ills such as abuse and criminal activity. The center contributes to data collection by monitoring the outcomes of its practice. Each community center is linked to other community centers, which in turn are linked to state and national centers. National centers are computer networked with centers throughout the world, all integrating and disseminating the most advanced knowledge. For example, based on this synthesis of information analysis, changes are made in pollution standards, or environmental alerts may be issued regarding solar radiation. Also, social trends are identified early on, and biopsychosociospiritual interventions are included in the criminal justice system. Because of the centralization of information and the use of artificial intelligence to help in sorting and coupling (comparing) information with the state-of-the-art knowledge bases, all interventions, including health, social, psychological, environmental, and criminal justice, are assessed for effectiveness and constantly improved.

The social wellness and health center has satellites in schools and places of work. The multiskilled professionals and volunteers in these satellites provide health screening and education, immunization, basic care, and case management with referrals to specialized services as needed. Volunteers in the schools include peer therapists, who are health resources for their classmates. These peer therapists receive special education and training along with mentoring from health professionals. They receive class credit for their work and practice their skills in hospitals and assisted-living centers as well as the schools. Volunteers in the workplace provide similar services for their peers, only they receive special education and mentoring that can be applied toward advanced degrees. In addition, the school- and business-based professionals coordinate parenting classes for families and prospective families as well as ongoing courses promoting wellness, self-esteem, and personal growth.

As Kaiser foretold, environmental health is a central focus: "Environmental health will be the first global issue on the planet earth. . . . If we do not stop fouling our nest, we die as a planet! Rule: if you don't manage a planet, you lose it. You want to see an unmanaged planet, tonight look up. If we continue our course of action, the earth will be a moon. If we don't take care, we will destroy our atmosphere, we will destroy our oceans, and we will destroy our life forms" (1991e, message 76). Environmental health is a pervasive component of the entire health system from the schools, workplace, and neighborhoods

to the federal government. People hold one another accountable for the health of the environment, in full recognition that
it is synonymous with human health.

Now health care is no longer patient-focused; it is patient-driven. The true center of the health care system lies within
the home via interactive computer networks. As Goldsmith
(1992) foretold, "The emergence of a capacity to predict and
manage disease pre-symptoms will provide a powerful set of new
tools not only to anticipate medical problems before they arise
but to empower individuals and families with knowledge to help
them improve their health status. . . . Each person will have [a]
genetic risk profile, identifying the major behavioral and environmental risk factors that must be controlled by the 'patient'
and his or her family to minimize disease risk" (p. 40).

Computer programs proliferate, allowing individuals to
enter symptoms and other data when ill. After data input, the
programs alert users to the need for further information, such
as testing through electromagnetic scanning, which can be performed by having the patient place a palm on a metal plate.
After the necessary data are obtained for diagnosis, diagnostic
options are presented with percentages of certainty. Users can
then access treatment options for each diagnosis along with their
costs and percentages of success. These treatment options include alternative methods such as massage, acupuncture, and
counseling approaches, as well as traditional medical and surgical interventions. Best therapy combinations and resources
for each therapy are also listed. These home computers can be
linked through subscription service to the social wellness and
health center, where information is constantly updated. When
needed, home and mobile technological units are available, as
most conditions can be treated in a home setting.

VR programs are also available for use in accessing healing potential; these vivid individualized scenes are tailored to
individuals and their needs. Freshley (1991, message 317) informs her readers: "Virtual reality has tremendous applications
in medical technology, especially in the area of diagnostic im-
aging. I see a future application in a Healing Healthcare environment where VR is used to create a virtual healing space

for the patient. I could request, as a patient, the opportunity to revisit some sacred space that brought me peace of mind. VR could take me there complete with sounds, scenes, and odors. I could walk through the space even as I lay in my bed. Or, I could use VR to explore a healing metaphor (Lee [Kaiser] mentions these as 'paths, gateways, tunnels' to greater being/ awareness)." VR is also used to enhance immune function through vivid holistic imagery and to decrease dependence on medications for the relief of pain. And it can be used for skills training. Individuals and practitioners can learn to perform medical procedure using virtual, interactive computer programs.

We have now developed an understanding of Era III health care. Health is defined as the expansion of consciousness, and illness episodes are viewed as invitations to a higher level of being. As Kaiser informs his readers, "Healing often occurs when the patient experiences a profound change in inner symbolism. New insights appear. A doorway to the future opens. Suddenly the patient's past and present take on new significance. Expanded meanings and purposes appear on the horizon of consciousness. Disease is no longer just an undesirable medical condition. It becomes a portal of initiation, a call to a higher level of being" (1991e, message 171). In this context, illness is explored as opportunity for learning and growth. The development of consciousness and human potential becomes a central role of health care. The caregiver is no longer doing but being, recast from custodian to counselor.

In Era III much thought is given to the hospital environment. The hospital is viewed as sacred in the sense that it is the place where we are born and die and experience our most vulnerable and transformative events. In this healing environment all aspects and dimensions of healing are attended to. The unique mythology and culture of the community are used in architecture as well as therapeutic interventions. Hospital design and architecture reveal an intention to provide comfort, nurturance, and safety. The healing power of nature is allowed and infused into the environment; waterfalls, windows with views, plants, and skylights are strategically placed. In addition, the hospital campus is designed to encourage patients and families to walk, talk, and quietly reflect in nature's cathedral.

The hospital incorporating Era III concepts acknowledges that the healing encounter has many dimensions. Key among these are the consciousness of the healer, the consciousness of the patient, and the relationship between the healer and the patient. Because of the importance of the unique being of the provider, providers are selected on the basis not only of their technical and clinical knowledge but also of their consciousness and commitment to learning and growth. Health care organizations provide ongoing seminars that facilitate personal growth and seminars focused on helping participants access their innate, natural healing potential. These seminars are open to providers, patients, and the community. Also, the unique cultural traditions of their service area are integrated into their learning programs.

The providers (doctors, nurses, housekeepers, dieticians, and others) are aware of their role as sacred "performers" who offer a life-transforming opportunity to patients. Great respect and healing intention occur in the relationship between provider and patient. The consciousness and belief system of the patient and family are assessed, and therapies are designed to promote their healing potential. For example, based on this assessment, the provider knows how much the patient and family want to participate in their own healing. Also, they know which methods to teach in eliciting the relaxation response: prayer, meditation, biofeedback, or simple breathing. In addition, they orchestrate the music and follow suggestions given by the surgery and recovery-room staff, and they may arrange for a medicine man, a pastor, a poet, or other volunteers to visit from the community.

Hospitals are only one component of the new health care system. As a result of biotechnological advances the need for acute care is decreased, and the focus is increasingly on trauma, serious infection, and the frail elderly. Hospitals provide this care through the collaborative efforts of multidisciplinary, self-directed teams. The management structure is circular and is designed to support the multidisciplinary team in providing patient-directed care.

With Era III health care, managers are mythmakers. Kaiser (1992) uses *myth* as conferring meaning upon or giving significance to. Managers' roles are spiritual ones, as they point the organization toward its meaning and keep it on track. These managers lead by the power of their vision and the clarity of their consciousness. They raise the consciousness of the organization and see the hospital as a system within systems. They promote the organization as a learning organization, where there are no mistakes, only opportunities for improvement and growth. Managers are philosophers, teachers, and guides. They are true mentors in the sense that they encourage their people to grow beyond them rather than being like them.

The organization is formed around its mission, vision, values, and standards. These are not just concepts but living and breathing realities, supported with agreements for interlocking accountability. Samuel (1991) describes this process: "Organizational success is a continuous process, not an event. It begins by clearly understanding the outcomes you desire for your customer, and translating those outcomes into operational language. Ultimately, each person must make the commitment to support continuous organization and team improvement, and be dedicated to self-improvement." With Era III health care, managers model healing in their relationships with others, creating safety and accountability. Likewise, team members are empowered to make a healing environment a reality for themselves and for their patients.

The Invitation

"I have been trying to think of the earth as a kind of organism, but it is no go. I cannot think of it this way. It is too big, too complex, with too many working parts lacking visible connections. The other night, driving through a hilly, wooded part of southern New England, I wondered about this. If not like an organism, what is it like, what is it most like? Then, satisfactorily for that moment, it came to me: it is most like a single cell" (Thomas, 1974, p. 4).

This is one view of what the new civilization in health care will look like. An important concept in systems thinking is that a change in one part of the system or the relationships between parts will affect the other parts and relationships. Health care itself is a system within systems, in the same way Thomas sees the earth as a cell within the universe. We acknowledge that when you change the health care system, you also affect the society and culture it is a part of. At the same time, when you change society, the government, or the environment, you change the nature of health care. Ultimately, though we may try, we are never truly in control of the system. It remains, ultimately, a mystery; we cannot know the vast, complex interactions of which we are a part. Everything is connected and interrelates with everything else.

Health care is not alone in its current need for change. Our families, our communities, our nations are searching for better ways of living and being with one another. As we saw with the learning society, our old methods of work and finding challenge and creativity in living are no longer available or relevant in an increasingly complex and technological society. People are searching for leadership and new structures that enhance living, learning, and healing.

This is the challenge we offer to health care. Patient-focused care is an obvious and important beginning; yet it is only a beginning. Who better than health care to pick up the mantle of healing? For what and for whom are we waiting? There are infinite possibilities for the new civilization, and we have presented but one view. Now we invite our readers to join us in defining the new era for health care. If you choose to do so, begin. That which has intention, compassion, vision, and action has magic.

Chapter 9

How You Can Become Involved

A journey of a thousand miles must begin with a single step.

Lao-tzu, 550 B.C.

In this book we presented our thesis that the survival of health care in this country depends on two key strategies: providing a holistic approach to healing, one that integrates body, mind, and spirit; and restructuring hospital operations in order to place patients and their needs at the center of health care's mission. We have explored these two strategies from multiple directions. First, we explored their impact on the bottom line in an environment of managed care, where economic survival lies in reducing costs by operating efficiently as well as by speeding patient healing and recovery. Then we presented several approaches that have proven to enhance healing and recovery and offered numerous strategies for their implementation. In addition, we presented a plan for operational restructuring, focused on patients and their needs. We then reviewed the effects of the traditional system on the health care team and presented some promising new models of care delivery. After showing how the physical environment can enhance or inhibit healing, we presented a vision for health care's future. Throughout, we have offered examples from pioneering hospitals across the country that have implemented these approaches. And, recognizing that our readers may want to pursue these approaches in depth, we have included a Resources Directory at the end of the book. This directory offers a number of resources ranging from books to places to visit.

238

Now that we have completed our journey through the many paths leading to a patient-centered and healing environment in hospitals, the reader may be wondering Where do I begin? or How can I become involved? Whether you are a health care consumer, a hospital administrator, a physician, a nurse, or any other member of the health care team, by reading this book you have taken the first step. In this chapter we will offer practical advice on how to continue the journey. Because this book has a wide audience all with different needs, we will separately address several broad categories of readers: health care consumers, hospital administrators, and nurses and other health care professionals. We end by giving suggestions for involving physicians in the process.

Health Care Consumers

As patients and other health care consumers you have more power than you may realize. The health care system cannot exist without you. Although there was a time when only the medical profession had all the knowledge and therefore made all the decisions, that time is clearly gone. Not only is your active involvement in your care the right thing to do, it is vital for your well-being. In Chapter Three we presented research that linked active patient and family involvement and enhanced healing, better health outcomes, fewer complications, and decreased cost because of shorter stays in the hospital.

We have to admit that health care as a whole has not done a good job of getting this kind of information to you. Yet nurses and physicians often wish patients would be active in their own health and recovery. For example, at a team-building session for new patient-centered care teams at St. Charles Medical Center, the surgical unit team developed a vision for care:

> The surgical floor team is recognized by our patients and their family as leaders in providing competent, excellent holistic healthcare. This care is delivered compassionately, professionally and with respect for the value of human diversity.

We employ open communication, working cooperatively to create and foster a nurturing environment that reflects trust, comfort and confidence. We recognize the need for and provide consistency of training and continuity of patient care with constant regard for our patients' physical, mental, spiritual and emotional needs. Our patients and their families feel valued and meeting their needs is our highest priority.

Afterward, they talked about how they were going to realize their vision. One nurse said, "I don't think patients know how important it is for them to be active participants in their care. Most patients think the patient role is a passive one and that the best thing is to let the nurses and doctors make the decisions and take care of them." After further discussion the team realized that health care providers have not taught the public how important it is for them to get actively involved. The group pointed out that this kind of information needs to get to people before they come to the hospital. "We need to do a better job of keeping our community updated on how important it is for them to be active participants in their own health care."

Patients today are seen as valuable customers by the hospital. In today's extremely competitive health care environment, each hospital is looking for ways to have a competitive edge. Most hospitals want to meet or exceed their patients' expectations.

Here are five practical ways to get involved. First, get to know your hospital's governing board and tell the members what you want from your local health care system. Every hospital has a board of directors, which is responsible for the overall direction of the hospital in meeting community needs.

Second, participate in hospital satisfaction surveys and focus groups. Most hospitals are interested in your impressions of their care and services and will use your information to improve their system. Be as forthright and honest as you can. Let them know what they can improve and let them know what they do well. Third, communicate your ideas and needs to hospital and physician-clinic administrators. Once again, most of these folks are eager to hear what you have to say. If they are not, talk directly to their board. Offer to speak at staff presentations if you are comfortable doing so. Hearing directly from their patients has the most effect in changing physician and staff behaviors. Also, as you may recall, it was the work of Angelica Thieriot, a patient who was shocked by her negative hospital experience, that started the patient-centered approach at Planetree, a model now being used by more and more hospitals throughout the world.

Fourth, form a consumer advocacy group. Consumers have a lot of power to change the system and groups of consumers have even more power. An excellent example of the collective power of the group is Mothers Against Drunk Driving. Through their collective efforts they have changed laws, saved lives, and affected the health of communities significantly. They have truly made a difference. If you want to get actively involved and are excited about the ideas in this book, you may want to use the book to start a discussion group. After you get started your group can decide whether it wants to be active on a local level or become a political-action group on the national level.

Fifth, be an active participant in making your health care decisions and in your care. This role may not feel comfortable at first. Many of us grew up believing that "doctor knows best" and may feel intimidated by the authoritarian figure of the physician. Believe me, the physician is just as human as you are. Often you will find that physicians are relieved to have patients take responsibility for their decisions and care. Be aware that you may not think of all your questions when you first get disturbing information; it is perfectly all right to say, "I need to think about this for awhile. Can I get back with you?"

Here are some more tips: Write your symptoms, concerns, and questions down in advance. If you feel nervous about talking to your doctor, have your nurse help you practice. Let both your doctor and nurse know your goals, what you want as a result of the treatment or hospital stay. Remember, you always have options. If you are not pleased with your treatment or care, let someone know as soon as possible. It's best if you tell the person directly. If that does not feel comfortable, tell the head nurse or the supervisor. I can almost guarantee they will be glad you let them know so they can improve service. Finally, you can ask for a second opinion. People in health care are used to this option now and recommend second opinions. It benefits them too; your belief and trust in your doctor or nurse have an affect on how well their treatment will work.

Hospital Administrators

These are challenging times for hospital administrators. Everyone knows hospitals have to change. But the questions of what, how, and when are not that easy to answer. Hospitals are in uncharted territory — uncharted territory with rough and choppy waters indeed. The downside is fear of the unknown and the upside is almost limitless opportunity. This book offers examples of how some hospitals are addressing this need to change; yet how do you begin? This is a personal decision for each hospital based on its developmental stage, community, and customers. One thing is certain: you cannot not change. To not change is to be dead in the water.

If you like some of the ideas in this book here are some suggestions for getting involved. First, check in with yourself. Do the ideas and approaches presented make sense to you? Do they get you excited? If they do, remember the words of Lathrop (1991, p. 21): "Few will challenge the goals of the patient-focused hospital. Many will question the means — telling us 'you can't get there from here.' The simple imperative is: We must get there, and here is the only place we can start. As long as we keep patients and common sense foremost in our minds, we will succeed."

Second, gather information. This book is a good start. You might also want to consider reading materials listed in the References for more details. In addition, the Resources Directory lists many excellent books, journals, organizations, associations, audiovisual resources, computer networks, consultants, and places to visit.

I particularly recommend the Healing Healthcare Network, the Healing Health Care Project (these are separate organizations), and talking to some of the consultants who are doing patient-focused restructuring. The Network publishes the *Healing Healthcare Network Newsletter,* which describes organizations that are incorporating healing approaches with conventional medical care, and offers the Healing Healthcare Network Computer Bulletin Board System (the BBS) and consultation services. The BBS serves as a primary means of networking for organizations that are furthering healing health care. Leland Kaiser, a prominent health care futurist, writes provocative editorials and a column on transformational leadership for the newsletter. The Healing Healthcare Project is a network of health care organizations, professionals, and community members. It offers networking opportunities and yearly symposiums for creatively addressing the problems in the American health care system.

Third, get others involved and committed. This involvement should start with top management, but it also must include middle management. A well-aligned management team is a key to the success of patient-focused care. It pays to take the time to get the management team fully informed and committed. For staff to get excited and involved without management's support is a set up for organizational conflict and stress.

Fourth, do an internal assessment. Where are you in relation to where you want to be? Some questions to consider:

Are you getting ready to embark on remodeling, renovation, or creating a new hospital? If so, you can integrate healing and patient-centered methods into your new design. Pat Linton, currently CEO of North Hawaii Community Hospital, is in this enviable position. He along with the hospital board members are involving the community in designing a "healing village," which is described in Chapter Nine. Also, Mark Scott, CEO of Mid-Columbia Medical Center, took advantage of the need for remodeling to implement a more homelike atmosphere as Mid-Columbia implemented Planetree concepts hospitalwide.

Is there a CQI process already in place? If so, integrate patient-focused concepts into it.

How do you compare on the elements of the patient-focused model presented in Chapter One? You may want to rate your organization on a scale of one to ten for each element, with ten being your vision for where you want to be.

Where can you begin right now in order to get immediate benefits? Immediate benefits will help with buy-in. St. Charles started with exception-based charting, which is guaranteed to free up time for patient care. Nearly everyone will agree that it makes sense to spend time nursing the patient instead of the chart.

What is the financial status of the hospital and what is the likelihood of success if you continue with the present mode of operation? Most of the hospitals undergoing patient-focused restructuring are in a stable financial state, although they predicted a high probability of financial disaster in the future if they continued with their previous course. Because the return on investment is long-range, the financial issue is a big one for hospitals. You may want to explore grants to fund the project.

Fifth, take key individuals on a site visit to show them a model that is up and running. Site visits are powerful ways to change people's minds. Not only can individuals see the process in action, but they can network with people who are doing it. These friendships are invaluable when it comes time for implementation and the inevitable questions arise. Sixth, attend relevant workshops and conferences.

Seventh, start a study group. For example, Sandy Heywood (1993), assistant to the president of Tucson Medical Center, started study groups around the Bill Moyer's television special "Healing and the Mind." In addition, TMC hosted a public forum with a panel of three physicians and two psychologists who reacted to the series and fielded questions from the audience. Eighth, develop a vision for what you want to create. Use the tension between what is and the vision to create the energy for change.

Ninth, appoint a person to spearhead the project. Although CEOs must generate the excitement and energy with their vision, it is unlikely they will have the time to keep the project moving forward. Jim Lussier, CEO of St. Charles Medical Center, appointed a director for its Healing Healthcare Project. The director is charged with further defining the project and process as well as coordinating activities. The plan is to bring the process into the organization's culture and dissolve the project as a separate entity after three years of intensive work.

Tenth, use consultants. Most hospitals look to consultants when undertaking major systems changes. You may want to review the guidelines for consultants in Chapter Four. Also, we have included a list of consultants for patient-focused restructuring in the Resources Directory.

Bill Adamski, founder of the ART of Living Institute, emphasizes that when you are changing an organization's paradigm you need someone from the outside to come in at regular intervals, someone who is sympathetic to what you are doing but not a part of the day-to-day politics of your organization. This person can hold the organization accountable for how they are doing and help the organization avoid being sucked into games of "good guy" versus "bad guy." The outside consultant can review how the process is going and see that people are not "beating up the leaders who are bringing about the change." It is characteristic of people going through organizational change to falter in their trust and belief in their own leaders. It helps to have an outsider come in to uncover the inevitable problems and facilitate their resolution.

Eleventh, develop champions. Many CEOs who have been through this process recommend identifying a few people representing key constituencies and gaining their support for your ideas. It helps to focus your energy on a few at first and then they can help get the word out and gain the support of others.

Twelfth, use pilot units. Once you have identified what you want to do, Kaiser (1991e) recommends trying the idea out in only one area at first. People who do not want to participate can choose to work elsewhere. The effects of the new design can be studied and refined before moving on to other areas. Of course, the administrator will need to weigh the economic benefits of moving on a larger scale. As models for patient-focused care are refined, they will be easier to implement on a large scale.

Nurses and Other Professionals

Health care is in transition. The chaos of these times makes fertile soil for growing new models of care delivery. The disciplines of nursing, social services, occupational therapy, physical therapy, respiratory therapy, and others all have a wonderful opportunity to join together and plan collaborative new models of care. The speed of the change has caught most professionals in health care by surprise, placing them in a reactive mode instead of a proactive mode — not that they all have not known that change has to happen.

Now is the time to begin collaborative planning using the tenets of patient-focused care and healing:

1. Make the patient the center of care. Services should be designed around the patient's needs.
2. Encourage active patient and family involvement and education.
3. Create a healing environment.
4. Provide continuity of care.
5. Use a holistic approach incorporating mind/body/spirit therapies.
6. Decentralize services to the patient-care unit whenever practical based on utilization. For example, if a group of patients requires eight hours of social services a day, make a social services person a permanent member of the team.
7. Become as flexible as possible through cross-training. Multiskilled practitioners are an absolute must. The days of widespread specialization are over. Specialization is not affordable in today's health care environment.
8. Leverage skills so that professionals are freed up to do what they are educated to do and lesser-skilled people help them with tasks.
9. Continuously study and improve quality. Eliminate waste and redundancy.

Let your manager know you want to explore how you can implement some or all of these tenets. Invite the manager to join you in forming a cross-functional planning group. Your manager may want to inform upper management before you begin. They may already be looking at these possibilities. If so, ask how you can become involved. If you get the go-ahead, think of your group as a think tank. Use these tenets as a starting point and begin creating your own model of patient-centered care. It is also wise to include someone who is a neutral observer of the process, someone who can help keep you on track. It will be natural for you to have blind spots and want to protect your usual way of doing things or your turf or territory. If you are already involved in patient-focused restructuring, use the methods of CQI to fine-tune and continually improve the quality of your care.

If this seems like an overwhelming task, start with one aspect that you feel excited about now. Be sure to analyze and develop your ideas before presenting them to management. Management is much more likely to accept your idea if you have thought it through and developed a plan to go with it. Here is a suggested outline for project management (Samuel, 1992):

1. Select your improvement goal.
2. Describe what you expect as an outcome.
3. Identify possible concerns.
4. Assign and do planning steps with target dates:
    a. Collect information. Study your process and method of doing things now. Use flow charts, time studies, and other such tools as needed.
    b. Analyze the situation.
    c. Brainstorm alternatives.
    d. Choose solutions.
    e. Prepare a presentation.
    f. Implement.
    g. Follow up implementation.
    h. Evaluate.

Nearly all the methods of enhancing healing in Chapter Three are within your scope of practice. You can begin doing them now. If you are not already well versed in adult education and relaxation skills, use the Resources Directory as a guide to references to increase your knowledge. For example, Davis, Eshelman, and McKay, *The Relaxation & Stress Reduction Workbook,* and Benson and Stuart, *The Wellness Book,* are excellent resources filled with practical information and exercises for learning these methods. Learn and practice these skills yourself before you teach them to patients. When you are teaching from a place of personal knowledge and familiarity, it is so much more meaningful to patients. You can practice and learn these skills on your own, but it is often easier to learn them with a group of people with whom you can share your experiences. People in your organization may already know these skills; they could facilitate your group. In addition, you can join some of the organizations listed, such as the American Holistic Nurses' Association.

In preparing for the future, nurses in particular need to prepare their educational map. Nursing has numerous entry levels to practice, from associate degree to doctorate. The breadth of nursing is one of its strengths, yet it can also be a weakness. Nurses need to be proactive now if they want to become involved in creating new roles for nursing in the community. These roles will focus on health, wellness, and human potential. Associate degree nurses are vital to the care of hospitalized patients, but nurses who wish to be community-based should begin now to pursue higher education. At the least you will need a bachelor's degree, and if you want to practice with more independence, a master's or nurse practitioner preparation will be required. Also, consider the value of the diversity offered by degrees in exercise physiology, counseling, or psychology. Nurses are ideal people for meeting the growing need for health-related counseling. Health care consumers trust nurses to teach, nurture, support, and advocate for them.

Physicians

One of the most prevalent questions in designing new approaches to care delivery, especially patient-focused care, is How do you get the physicians involved? Physicians, too, have been caught by the speed of change demanded by our consumers. By and large their reaction has been reactive and their role more as spectator than as active participant in these new changes. Yet physicians have a great deal of influence on patient-focused care. New models will not succeed unless physicians are involved.

In order to shed some light on this important issue we

draw on our own learning as well as the work of Gerteis, Daley, Delbanco, and Edgman-Levitan (1993). One of the coauthors, Thomas Delbanco, through his experience as a practicing internist for twenty years and his research at the Picker/Commonwealth Program for Patient-Centered Care, offers a useful review of factors influencing physician behaviors and strategies for physician involvement. This research involved 6,455 patients and approximately 2,000 care partners selected randomly from sixty-two hospitals across the nation. This study found that patients view physicians with a large range of emotion, ranging from respect and awe to fear and mistrust. They also have a variety of perceptions of the physician's role, from captain of the ship to subordinate. According to Delbanco, more than 10 percent of the patients interviewed noted physicians talking in front of them as if they were not there, and more than 15 percent felt no single physician was in charge of their care.

Here are some attributes of physicians as a group:

1. Physicians view hospitals as competitors or employers. This is a shift in view that started in the late 1960s and early 1970s, when hospitals started hiring physicians as primary caregivers in immediate-care centers, clinics, and other areas.

2. Physicians believe they are patient-centered. They are eager to please their patients. At the same time, they feel pinched by time constraints, encroaching technology, bureaucratic demands for reimbursement, and a litigious society.

3. Physicians are worried about the doctor/patient relationship and the faltering image of physicians. They are concerned about "doctor shopping" and the fact that more and more patients question their doctors' judgment and seek second opinions. They worry about attracting and retaining patients as evidenced by the proliferation of marketing strategies directed to both patients and third-party payers.

4. Physicians respond to data. Much of the emphasis of their education is on the importance of drawing on data in making decisions.

5. Physicians thrive on specifics and abhor generalities.

6. Physicians would rather get feedback directly from patients than from other health care providers or administrators.
7. Close colleagues hesitate to find fault with one another.
8. Physicians rely on hospital staff, including residents and interns, for quality care. They recognize that patients perceive their care as a single experience. Doctors reap the benefits of good hospital care and pay the price for bad hospital care.
9. Physicians want to give top-quality clinical care.
10. Physicians carry a great deal of responsibility. They not only work long hours but frequently worry about their patients when away from work.

Here are some strategies for involving physicians. First, identify and develop champions, preferably opinion leaders. It may be wise, at first, to focus your efforts on a few supporters who in turn can help reach the rest of their colleagues. Second, use physicians to teach physicians. Doctors learn best from doctors. Third, provide physicians with specific data from their patients. These data can be from patient focus groups or patient surveys. If patient surveys are used, they need to provide specific information, identifying specific physicians.

Fourth, look for the "teachable moment." Watch for times when a group of doctors complain about patient care or a hospital problem. Then get them involved by challenging them to solve the problem. Physicians enjoy challenges. Take this opportunity to provide "just in time training" for using some of the specific tools of operational restructuring or TQM. Use the momentum of patient-focused restructuring as an entry to CQI.

Fifth, institute CQI or TQM. Using these systems means using statistical data and focusing on the system versus pointing fingers. Dr. Brent C. James (as cited by Geber, 1992) of Intermountain Healthcare Inc., a Salt Lake City–based chain of twenty-four hospitals that began TQM in 1986, uses statistical data to generate discussion about the methods doctors use to treat illnesses or perform procedures. "Doctors," James says, "are driven by a desire to deliver the best possible care to patients, and they don't want to be out of step with their colleagues.

If it can be statistically proven to them that superior care can be delivered at less cost, they will rarely resist" (p. 31).

Geber offers another example. At Atlanta West Paces Ferry Hospital, a group of physicians, midwives, and nurses was studying their Caesarean rate of just over 22 percent. They discovered one of the major causes was that the pregnant women's own mothers did not realize how medicine has changed since they gave birth. The mothers were convinced that vaginal births would be dangerous for their daughters. Faced with a patient who feared vaginal birth, the average physician simply acquiesced. The hospital reduced the C-section rate to 16 percent by offering classes for pregnant mothers and their mothers. As the team continued their work, they found that when labor stalled and the drug pitocin was given to advance labor, C-section rates increased to 23 percent. As a result of this finding, they matched their hospital against hospitals in Denmark that have the lowest C-section rates in the world. The team found that by giving mothers warm baths and encouraging them to walk, they were able to lower the C-section rate to less than 5 percent. Now, the overall C-section rate is below 10 percent, one of the lowest in the nation.

Sixth, provide physicians with aggregate data about their patients. A good example of the effectiveness of this kind of data is offered by Gerteis, Daley, Delbanco, and Edgman-Levitan (forthcoming, pp. 382–383) in describing how findings from their study changed a physician's behavior.

> He learned further that many of these patients [chronically ill] recalled spending less than five minutes with the doctor in preparation for discharge. In response, the doctor changed his behavior. Concentrating in particular on his patients with chronic illness, he spent more time with them on the day of discharge, addressing in detail what they might or might not do once back home. While this effort led him to spend some extra time on the hospital wards, he believes the net impact has been to save time. Indeed, he appears delighted by his impres-

sion that he has decreased morbidity in several patients and may well have prevented readmission for
some. He receives fewer phone calls from patients
seeking clarification once home.

Seventh, provide physicians with research documenting
the efficacy of patient-focused care. Physicians need hard data
to convince them that communication and attention to the needs
of the whole person are not just "frills" that pale beside the need
for biomedical care. You may want to use some of the research
cited in Chapter Three. Much of this research is printed outside of the journals that physicians usually read. Delbanco recommends the use of annotated bibliographies, clinical reviews,
and other methods of continuing education to help physicians
(Gerteis, Daley, Delbanco, and Edgman-Levitan, forthcoming).

Eighth, be aware that physicians will respond to a focused
effort to improve the quality of patient care if they are invited
to work on challenging problems in a collaborative way. Ninth,
advocate to enhance medical school education and training by
including communication, relational skills, and other patient-
centered and healing dimensions in the curriculum. Harvard
Medical School is now teaching physicians relaxation skills for
use by themselves and with their patients. Other medical schools
are adding programs in which physicians are required to spend
time as hospitalized patients to learn about care from the patient's point of view. Delbanco recommends that because the
interpersonal aspects of care affect patient outcomes, they should
be both explored and modeled during teaching rounds (Gerteis, Daley, Delbanco, and Edgman-Levitan, forthcoming).

Tenth, use computer software that enhances patient participation and frees physicians' time for human contact. Some of
these tools are listed in the Resources Directory. Eleventh, use
educational material, such as interactive video, printed material, and audiotapes to enhance patient and family learning.
Twelfth, streamline and enhance systems to allow physicians time
for patient contact. For example, initiate an automated patient
record on which patients and families can review the physician's
observations and impressions and enter their own as well. Thir-

teenth, set up reward and recognition programs for physicians. Doctors are people too. Recognition in employee newsletters or from patients means a lot to physicians.

Finally, Delbanco offers these suggestions for enhancing the physician/patient relationship: Use patients as teachers for physicians and hospital staff. Record pivotal conversations with patients and families and give the tape to the patient. Send patients written summaries of interactions. Physicians can be made aware of these suggestions.

Closing

Transforming health care is everyone's business. No one group or individual can do it alone. It requires a collaborative effort. President Bill Clinton said in his 1993 Inaugural Address, "Today we pledge an end to the era of deadlock and drift — and a season of American renewal has begun." We live in a time when people say that the cost of health care is crippling our country, threatening to bankrupt businesses small and large. To renew health care we must be bold; we must have the courage of our conviction that the purpose of health care is to enhance the healing and wellness of the people we serve. It is not an easy task to change the form of structures already in place. It would be easier to start anew, with a clean slate. Yet, we have nowhere to begin but where we are. Again, President Clinton urges us to "take more responsibility, not only for ourselves and our families but for our communities and our country."

We have offered our vision for health care's future and we have described the creative and bold efforts of numerous hospitals throughout our country that are taking responsibility for creating new approaches, new systems of care delivery. It is a process without end. We must recognize that change is a part of life, and every model and method we create must be continually evaluated and improved. We must join together — hospital administrators, health care professionals, physicians, community leaders, and citizens — to recognize that we need each other to create a health care system that truly cares for the health of our people.

Resources Directory

This directory contains some of the resources we have used in developing our perceptions of health care that heals as well as cures. Also, to enrich our list we have included resources noted in Sasenick (1992a, 1992b) as well as in the *Healing Health-care Network Newsletter.*

Books

Achterberg, J. *Imagery in Healing.* Boston: Shambhala, 1985.

This is a classic in our view and required reading for anyone interested in imagery. Achterberg provides an in-depth overview of the imagination as healer, including its roots in shamanism and in Western medicine through Aesclepius, Aristotle, Galen, and Hippocrates. She follows the golden thread of imagery to modern times and its use on the frontiers of health in the field of immunology.

Benson, H., and Stuart, E. *The Wellness Book: The Comprehensive Guide to Maintaining Health and Treating Stress-Related Illness.* New York: Carol Publishing Group, 1992.

This book is designed for patients as a guide to the behavioral-medicine clinics at the New England Deaconess Hospital in Boston. It is the result of twenty-five years of scientific research and clinical practice at the Harvard Medical School and three of its teaching hospitals. Each chapter is designed to help the reader develop important mind/body skills and attitudes for wellness.

Blayney, K. (ed.). *Healing Hands: Customizing Your Health Team for Institutional Survival.* Battle Creek, Mich.: W. K. Kellogg Foundation, 1992.

This book offers approaches to employing and training multiskilled health care workers and provides information on their influence on quality and cost-effectiveness. To order a free copy, call (800) 367-3465.

Borysenko, J. *Minding the Body: Mending the Mind.* Reading, Mass.: Addison-Wesley, 1987.

Borysenko offers her readers a personal journey of healing as she shares her own story as well as the stories of some of the patients she worked with at the Mind/Body Clinic in Boston. The book is easy to read and informative.

Cohen, U., and Day, K. *Holding On to Home: Designing Environments for People with Dementia.* Baltimore, Md.: Johns Hopkins University Press, March 1991.

This book offers therapeutic design tips for people with dementia.

Davis, M., Eshelman, E., and McKay, M. *The Relaxation & Stress Reduction Workbook.* Oakland, Calif.: New Harbinger, 1988.

This is a practical, easy-to-use workbook for teaching relaxation and stress reduction. The exercises can be taught by anyone. The basic premise of this book is that the benefits of relaxation and stress-reduction methods can be realized only after they have been practiced regularly over a period of time. Intellectual understanding is of little value without firsthand experience. The authors also offer a companion teacher's guide.

Dossey, B., Keegan, L., Guzzetta, C., and Kolmeier, L. *Holistic Nursing: A Handbook for Practice.* Gaithersburg, Md.: Aspen, 1988.

This is a great resource book for holistic practitioners. It offers information, exercises, and research on practices such as imagery and therapeutic touch.

Hoffman, L. *Foundations of Family Therapy: A Conceptual Framework for Systems Change.* New York: Basic Books, 1981.

Although this book is written for family therapists, we found it an excellent resource for understanding systems theory and systems change from a humanistic point of view.

Holland, J., and Rowland, J. (eds.). *Handbook of Psychooncology: Psychological Care of the Patient with Cancer.* New York: Oxford University Press, 1990.

We recommend this book as a comprehensive resource for the psychological care of cancer patients. It is a rich source for an overview of psychological and social adaptation, psychiatric disorders, central-nervous-system complications, ethical issues, and relevant research.

Mitchell, J., and Bray, G. *Emergency Services Stress: Guidelines for Preserving the Health and Careers of Emergency Services Personnel.* Englewood Cliffs, N.J.: Prentice-Hall, 1990.

This book offers an easy-to-follow guide for doing critical-incident stress debriefings. It is easy to read and comprehensive in the coverage of the topic.

Pelletier, K. *Holistic Medicine.* New York: Delta, 1979.

Pelletier is a leader in holistic medicine. This book is an excellent resource for those who want to know more about this area of research and study.

Rossi, E. *The Psychobiology of Mind-Body Healing.* New York: W. W. Norton, 1986.

This fantastic book offers an excellent description of the mind/body connection. Rossi, a Jungian psychotherapist, is one of the outstanding practitioners of hypnosis in our time. The book is fairly easy to understand and gives an excellent introduction to key concepts like state-dependent learning, information transduction, hypnosis, and psychoneuroimmunology.

Siegel, B. *Love, Medicine and Miracles.* New York: HarperCollins, 1987.

This well-known book describes the author's findings in his work with exceptional cancer patients. The book is rich with patients' stories and leaves the reader with a sense of renewed hope. Often, I give it to patients to read.

Journals

Aesclepius. Aesclepius is the newsletter of the National Symposium on Healthcare Design. Published three times a year, it offers information on how design of the physical environment affects therapeutic outcomes and on the current activities of the Symposium. Subscribe by calling (510) 370-0345.

The Futurist. This journal provides information from futurists, who watch trends and anticipate future events. It is published by the World Future Society, 7910 Woodmont Avenue, Suite 450, Bethesda, Maryland 20814. The editor is Cynthia Wagner.

Healing. This official journal of the Healing Health Care Project is dedicated to creating a new vision of the healing relationship as a mutual effort. It is published four times a year by the Health Communication Research Institute, Inc., Suite 105, 1050 Fulto Avenue, Sacramento, California 95825. The executive editor is Marlene von Friederichs-Fitzwater.

Healing Healthcare Network Newsletter. This quarterly newsletter promotes the healing aspect of health care. It describes organizations that incorporate healing approaches into their conventional medical care. Ongoing sections discuss high-touch healing, healing resources, healing communities, research, and healing design. Leland R. Kaiser, Ph.D., writes provocative editorials and a column on transformational leadership. The newsletter is published by Kaiser & Associates, P.O. Box 339, Brighton, Colorado 80601. Phone: (303) 659-2446.

Healthcare Forum Journal. This journal explores current issues in health care. It is published bimonthly by The Healthcare Forum, 830 Market Street, San Francisco, California 94102. The editor is Susan J. Anthony.

Holistic Medicine. This is the official journal of the American Holistic Medical Association and Foundation. Published six times a year, it covers relevant topics and the activities of the Association. American Holistic Medical Association and Foundation, 2002 Eastlake Avenue East, Seattle, Washington 98102. The editor is Gurudhan Khalsa.

Journal of Healthcare Design. This journal documents the proceedings of the annual National Symposium on Healthcare Design. It is available by calling (415) 370-0345.

The Noetic Sciences Review. This is the journal of the Institute of Noetic Sciences. It is published quarterly by the Institute of Noetic Sciences, 475 Gate Five Road, Suite 300, Sausalito, California 94965. The editor is Barbara McNeill.

Organizations and Associations

The American College of Physician Executives. This national organization of physicians is committed to increasing both skills in management and knowledge about the physician's role in management. It offers ongoing programs on personal fulfillment, professional growth and recognition, and management education. The College holds a seat in the American Medical Association House of Delegates and is recognized as a specialty organization by the American Medical Association. For more information, write to The American College of Physician Executives, Suite 200, 4890 West Kennedy Boulevard, Tampa, Florida 33609-2575. Phone: (800) 562-8088.

The American Holistic Medical Association. This organization is dedicated to bringing healing to medical practice. It describes its goal as "to facilitate healing of body, mind and spirit through health promotion, education, conventional and complementary forms of medical treatment." It also holds regular conferences and publishes a newsletter, *Holistic Medicine*. For more information, write to The American Holistic Medical Association, 2002 Eastlake Avenue East, Seattle, Washington 98102. Phone: (206) 322-6842.

American Holistic Nurses' Association. This association is dedicated to guiding the contemporary nurse in a challenging role. The Association defines the holistic approach as addressing the body, mind, and spirit. It offers many conferences and workshops to help nurses keep abreast of high-touch therapies, and it publishes current research in the *Journal of Holistic Nursing*. For more information, write to American Holistic Nurses' Association, Suite 511, 205 St. Louis Street, Springfield, Missouri 65806. Phone: (417) 864-5160.

ART of Living Institute. This institute uses the ARTWorks paradigm developed by Bill Adamski. Adamski offers ART of Living Core Courses, healing programs for hospital employees, physicians, and patients. The core course is a powerful way to help people become accountable for themselves and to take charge of their personal/relational and organizational vision. The ontological approach of the ART of Living Institute also underlies the philosophy of the integrated medical unit at Washoe Medical Center. For more information, write to ART of Living Institute, P.O. Box 160603, Sacramento, California 95816. Phone: (916) 676-3931.

The Center for Attitudinal Healing. The Center offers services to assist children, youth, and adults with life-threatening illness. It supplements traditional health care through enhancing the quality of living. It offers support for people with long-term illnesses, their caregivers, the disabled, and people dealing with bereavement. It also offers specialized training programs and workshops for health care professionals as well as consultation about various topics such as health/wellness management. For more information, write to The Center for Attitudinal Healing, 19 Main Street, Tiburon, California 94920. Phone: (415) 435-5022.

The Center for Knowledge Coupling. This nonprofit organization's purpose is to accelerate the development and availability of the Problem-Knowledge Coupler System. This medical problem-solving and decision-support software was created and developed by Lawrence Weed, developer of the Problem-Oriented Medical Record. This system couples (compares) each patient's problem-specific profile with the literature (knowledge). The result is neither a computer diagnosis nor a cookbook recipe for management. It is a powerful guidance system that provides a shortcut from the patient's problem to knowledge about the problem. This tool can be used by both patients and physicians. For more information, contact Vergil Slee, M.D., 16 Udoque Court, Brevard, North Carolina 28712. Phone: (704) 884-6508.

Commonweal. This not-for-profit center for service in and research on the area of health and human ecology is an excellent resource for material on complementary treatment methods, both adjunctive and alternative. The Institute for the Study of Health and Illness at Commonweal provides opportunities for physicians, psychologists, and other health professionals working with life-threatening illnesses to learn innovative ways to treat the whole person. In addition, the Commonweal Projects in Patient-Centered Medicine offer activities supporting the development of patient-centered medicine and health care. For more information, write to Commonweal, P.O. Box 316, Bolinas, California 94924. Phone (415) 868-0970.

The Elisabeth Kübler-Ross Center. This nonprofit organization is dedicated to the promotion of the concept of unconditional love as an attainable ideal. Its purpose is to spread knowledge and understanding of this concept along with its underlying premises: as we accept full responsibility for all of our feelings, thoughts, actions, and choices, and as we, in a safe environment, release negative emotions that we repressed in the past, we can live free, happy, and loving lives, at peace with ourselves and others. They offer life, death, and transition workshops, follow-up intensive workshops, and training programs. For more information, write to The Elisabeth Kübler-Ross Center, South Route 616, Head Waters, Virginia 24442. Phone: (703) 396-3441.

Environmental Design Research Association, Inc. The purpose of this international, interdisciplinary organization is to advance the art and science of environmental-design research. The Association is concerned with the effect of environments on family organization, recovery of patients, and worker productivity. Using environmental-design research, it seeks to improve understanding of the interrelationships of people, their buildings, and the natural environment. Through this understanding environments can be created that are responsive to human needs. For more information, write to Environmental Design Research Association, Inc., P.O. Box 24083, Oklahoma City, Oklahoma 73124. Phone: (405) 843-4863.

The Foundation for Hospital Art, Inc. This foundation provides art at no cost to not-for-profit/charity hospitals and nursing homes. For more information, write to The Foundation for Hospital Art, Inc., 230 Hillswick Court, Atlanta, Georgia 30328. Phone: (404) 393-2931.

Healing Healthcare Network. The Healing Healthcare Network is an association of organizations committed to developing health care that heals as well as cures. The Network publishes the *Healing Healthcare Network Newsletter* and serves as a resource for people seeking information on topics like complementary medicine, patient-centered care, psychoarchitecture, light and sound in health care environments, therapeutic touch, massage therapy, psychoneuroimmunology. For more information, write to Healing Healthcare Network, P.O. Box 339, Brighton, Colorado 80601. Phone: (303) 659-2446.

Healing Health Care Project. The Healing Health Care Project is a network of health care organizations, professionals, and members of the community who are creatively addressing the problems of the American health care system. The project is committed to systems, protocols, and partnerships that allow for the empowerment of the whole person. It offers yearly symposiums and ongoing opportunities for networking and learning for members. For more information, write to Healing Health Care Project, 1050 Fulton Avenue, Suite 105, Sacramento, California 95825. Phone: (916) 483-7301.

Healing Healthcare Systems. Susan Mazer and Dallas Smith have developed and produced audio/video programming (music and ambient images) specifically for health care facilities. Such programming contributes to the creation of healing environments and affects therapeutic objectives. They also offer a training and development strategy to empower the staff to participate intentionally in the design of the clinical environment. Their strategy has three components: Music-in-Residence: an environmental intervention; Music: A Life-Altering Decision: an experiential workshop for health care professionals; and Music-in-Action follow-up seminars: small-group workshops. For more information, write to Healing Healthcare Systems, Box 17511, South Lake Tahoe, California 96150. Phone: (916) 541-0901. Fax: (916) 541-1611.

Institute for Music, Health & Education. Don Campbell, founder and director of the Institute, is a pioneer in the therapeutic use of sound and psychoacoustics in health care. For more information, write to Institute for Music, Health & Education, P.O. Box 1244, Boulder, Colorado 80306. Phone: (303) 443-8484.

Institute of Noetic Sciences. This organization was founded in 1973 to support research and education on human consciousness. Its purposes are to broaden knowledge of the nature and potential of mind and consciousness, and to apply that knowledge to enhance the quality of life. For more information, write to Institute of Noetic Sciences, Suite 300, 475 Gate Five Road, P.O. Box 909, Sausalito, California 94966-0909.

Institute on Aging and the Environment. This organization's mission is to enhance older persons' quality of life. Their mission is accomplished through research, educational programs, innovative programming, and design practices that are sensitive to aging persons' concerns. For more information, write to Professor Uriel Cohen, Director, Institute on Aging and the Environment, School of Architecture and Urban Planning, University of Wisconsin, P.O. Box 413, Milwaukee, Wisconsin 53201. Phone: (414) 229-6481.

InterHealth. InterHealth is an alliance of Christian health organizations dedicated to improving members' business performance while enhancing Christian values. InterHealth provides interrelated services to members in the areas of research, knowledge exchange, project work, and advocacy. It also forms partnerships that link members with other organizations in order to create new opportunities or advance similar goals. For more information, write to InterHealth, Suite 233 North, 2550 University Avenue West, St. Paul, Minnesota 55114-1052. Phone: (612) 646-5574.

Leadership Dynamics, Inc. Leadership Dynamics offers training in personal development and communication skills that result in increased energy and resources for organizations. As people learn to lead skillfully and to contribute fully to their work, organizations gain effective teams, good decisions, and improved morale. Leadership Dynamics training focuses on maximizing the human element in organizations. For more information, write to Leadership Dynamics, Inc., 40 East Broadway, Eugene, Oregon 97401. Phone: (503) 683-6343.

The Milton H. Erickson Foundation, Inc. This organization strives to promote dialogue among schools of psychotherapy. To accomplish this goal it organizes an international congress every three years. It also offers many educational and training workshops. For more information, write to The Milton H. Erickson Foundation, Inc., 3606 North 24th Street, Phoenix, Arizona 85016. Phone: (602) 956-6196.

Mind/Body Medical Institute. Herbert Benson, authority on the relaxation response, started this organization. The therapies used at the Institute are a result of more than twenty-five years of scientific research and clinical practice at the Harvard Medical School and three of its major teaching hospitals. Its programs consist of outpatient, interdisciplinary, nonpharmacologic group interventions for the treatment of conditions caused by stress. Patients include those with cancer, chronic pain, insomnia, infertility, cardiac problems, AIDS/ARC/HIV+, and general stress-related disorders. The Institute offers clinical training in behavioral medicine and consultation for Mind/Body Clinic affiliation. For more information, write to Mind/Body Medical Institute, New England Deaconess Hospital, 185 Pilgrim Road, Boston, Massachusetts 02215. Phone: (617) 732-9525.

The National Institute for the Clinical Application of Behavioral Medicine. This organization offers conferences on advances in behavioral medicine. For more information, write to The National Institute for the Clinical Application of Behavioral Medicine, Box 523, Mansfield Center, Connecticut 06250. Phone: (203) 429-2238.

National Resource Center on Worksite Health Promotion. A cooperative initiative of the Washington Business Group on Health, the Office of Disease Prevention and Health Promotion, and the U.S. Public Health Service, the Center has as its mission work-site health promotion and disease-prevention programs and policies. This organization serves as a forum for the discussion of critical issues in work-site health promotion, and it is a resource for identifying innovative programs and practices that meet employer and employee needs. For more information, write to National Resource Center on Worksite Health Promotion, Suite 800, 777 North Capitol Street NE, Washington, D.C. 20002. Phone: (202) 408-9320.

National Symposium on Healthcare Design, Inc. Dedicated to improving the quality of the health care environment, the

Symposium has a worldwide, multidisciplinary audience. It also publishes *Aesclepius*. For more information, write to National Symposium on Healthcare Design, Inc., 4550 Alhambra Way, Martinez, California 94553-4406. Phone: (510) 370-0345.

Nurse Healers–Professional Associates, Inc., Cooperative. This international network of health professionals facilitates the exchange of research findings, teaching strategies, and information on new developments in clinical practice related to the exploration and expansion of healing modalities. Within this cooperative context the human being is viewed as a complex, dynamic whole, and healing is seen as the means of restoring and maintaining the integrity of mind, body, and spirit. For more information, write to Nurse Healers–Professional Associates, Inc., Cooperative, Suite 3399, 234 Fifth Avenue, New York, New York 10001.

Audiovisual Resources

Brighton Books. This publisher offers all of Leland R. Kaiser's many works. These works include books as well as audiotapes and videotapes. An excellent videotape to begin with is *The Hospital as a Healing Community.* For more information, write to Brighton Books, P.O. Box 339, Brighton, Colorado 80601. Phone: (303) 659-8815 or (800) 223-5999.

Dr. Know, The Medical Media Store. This store carries over 2,000 videos on health, relaxation, and medical procedures. It also provides a computerized health reference system, Dr. Know On-Line. This user-friendly system provides easy access to periodical indices, abstracts, article summaries, articles, and references from encyclopedias and medical books. For more information, write to Dr. Know, 803 Congress Street, Portland, Maine 04102. Phone: (800) 877-3112.

Hospital Video Theater Laff Therapy. This services offers a rotating library of videotapes of comedy performers. For more information, call (800) 950-4248.

New Dimensions Radio. This radio program offers interviews with cutting-edge thinkers and state-of-the-art practitioners about healing methods. For a catalog, write to New Dimensions Foundation, P.O. Box 410510, San Francisco, California 94141. Phone: (415) 563-8899.

Osborn Healthcare Communications. This is an innovative computerized, televised, and individualized patient and staff education system. For more information, write to Osborn Healthcare Communications, Suite 585, 3401 West End Avenue, Nashville, Tennessee 37203. Phone: (800) 726-1496.

Computer Network

Healing Healthcare Network Computer Bulletin Board System (BBS). The BBS is a primary means of networking for organizations that are furthering healing health care. They use this medium to share projects, learnings, and research both among themselves and with specialists in particular areas. If you want to participate or would like more information, contact John Carlson, Executive Director, Healing Healthcare Network, at (303) 659-2446.

Consultants

Healing Health Care and Patient-Centered Care

BKB Associates. Dr. Betty Bell, R.N., D.N.S., combines her extensive management and organization-development experience to provide consultation services and education programs to health care professionals and organizations seeking individual and organizational transformation. Bell assists her clients in designing and implementing vision-based change that incorporates healing, personal power, and partnership. Her services result in the creation of powerful and effective teams committed to bringing about healing through personal commitment and ownership. For more information, write to BKB Associates, 4109 Scranton Circle, Carmichael, California 95608. Phone: (916) 971-1169.

Consulting Services Network (CSN). CSN is a national network of independent speakers and health care consultants organized into seven topical groups. Members of the Healing Healthcare Group and Healthcare Facilities Design Group are dedicated to assisting hospitals in implementing healing health care technologies. For detailed information about the members of these two groups, contact Kevin Kaiser, executive director. For more information, write to Consulting Services Network, P.O. Box 339, Brighton, Colorado 80601. Phone: (303) 659-7311.

The Creative Connection. This is a network of innovative professionals committed to enhancing the health and well-being of society through the design of environments with a healing intention. These professionals design physical and relational spaces that support the client, staff, and organization. This support is provided through the use of simple tools such as art, color, lighting, stained glass, plants, aroma, sound, water, and the support of individual and group relationships in the physical space. For more information, write to Diane M. Bush, R.N., M.P.H., The Creative Connection, 3281 Mountain Lake Drive, Pollock Pines, California 95726. Phone: (916) 644-0884.

IMPAQ Organizational Improvement Systems. IMPAQ is dedicated to the healing of organizations through the transformation of reactive management into proactive leadership. As the originator of "accountability-based" systems and training, IMPAQ consultants assist organizations in creating and nurturing a true continuous-quality-improvement culture based on accountability and support. They specialize in planning for and creating self-directed, cross-functional, patient-centered-care teams. They also assist organizations in management development and in the implementation of customer service necessary for supporting the change to a culture of commitment, trust, integrity, and continuous learning/improvement. For more information, write to IMPAQ, West Coast Division, Suite 3, 1744 West Katella, Orange, California 92667. Phone: (714) 744-8941.

Komras & Associates, Inc. Komras & Associates is dedicated to improving management performance and organization development in health care organizations. The company offers management training programs and a unique video-based assessment tool for measuring management competence. Komras offers presentations and workshops on patient-focused care, empowerment, self-esteem, and thinking skills. For more information, write to Komras & Associates, Inc., Suite 206, 1515 North Warson Rd., St. Louis, Missouri 63132. Phone: (314) 429-5450.

Lemmon Associates. Don McKahan, architect and planner, works with hospitals to create healing health care architecture. Leland Kaiser and McKahan have produced a video, *Healing by Design: Creating Therapeutic Environments for Healthcare,* available through Brighton Books. For more information, write to Lemmon Associates, 1307 Stratford Court, Del Mar, California 92014. Phone: (619) 259-9244.

Planetree. This consumer health organization advocates for patient-centered health care. It assists hospitals in changing from being intimidating, impersonal institutions to being places of nurturance, education, and healing. For more information, write to California Pacific Medical Center, 2040 Webster Street, San Francisco, California 94115. Phone: (415) 923-3696.

Patient-Focused Restructuring

Anderson Consulting
Ned Troup, Partner
2100 One PPG Place
Pittsburgh, Pennsylvania 15222
(412) 232-7071

APM, Incorporated
David Bellaire, Principal
One Bush Street, Suite 400
San Francisco, California 94104
(415) 362-8266

Booz, Allen Health Care, Inc.
J. Philip Lathrop, Vice President
225 West Wacker Drive
Chicago, Illinois 60606-1228
(312) 578-4702

Coopers & Lybrand
Charles C. Gabbert, Principal
350 South Grand Avenue
Los Angeles, California 90071
(213) 356-6449

Ernst & Young
Sandra Wisener, Partner
2001 Ross Avenue, Suite 2800
Dallas, Texas 75201
(214) 979-1720

First Consulting Group
Warren Guillett, Vice President
Management & Clinical Consulting Services
27950 Orchard Lake Road, Suite 101
Farmington Hills, Michigan 48334
(313) 350-1705

Hay Management Consultants
Katherine W. Vestal, Ph.D.
National Director/Work Restructuring
12801 North Central Expressway
Dallas, Texas 75243-1731
(214) 934-6800

Senn-Delaney Leadership Group
John Childress, President and C.E.O.
4510 East Pacific Coast Highway, Suite 300
Long Beach, California 90804
(312) 494-3398
(Specializes in executive leadership training)

Places to Visit

Bishop Clarkson Memorial Hospital. Mitch Galloway, Patient-Focused-Care Coordinator, 44th and Dewey Avenue, Omaha, Nebraska 68105-1018. Phone: (402) 552-3588. Bishop Clarkson, a 320-bed tertiary hospital, opened its pilot unit in the summer of 1990 and planned to complete hospitalwide restructuring within three years. Patient-focused operating units now in place are oncology/gastrointestinal, kidney/genitourinary, obstetrics, cardiopulmonary, and orthopedics/neurology. Bishop Clarkson Memorial is part of the six-hospital, patient-focused restructuring consortium led by Booz, Allen Health Care, Inc. and is instituting continuous quality improvement and self-directed work teams.

Lakeland Regional Medical Center. Dennis Shortridge, Executive Vice President/C.O.O., P.O. Box 95448, Lakeland, Florida 33804. Phone: (813) 687-1195. Lakeland, an 897-bed full-service hospital, is a pioneer in patient-focused restructuring. It began the process in 1988. In 1989 it opened its first patient-focused general surgery unit. By December 1990 the unit expanded to include another wing, with ENT, vacular, oral, plastic surgery, and neurosurgery patients. Following this, in 1992, a new forty-eight-bed urological and gynecological/oncology surgery unit was restructured. Envisioned in the future are five operating units, or "minihospitals," that will encompass the entire organization after the completion of a five-year development plan.

Mid-Columbia Medical Center. Mark Scott, President, 1700 East 19th Street, The Dalles, Oregon 97058. Phone: (503) 296-7273. A forty-nine-bed, rural, tertiary referral center, Mid-Columbia is the first to adopt the Planetree model hospitalwide. It offers everyone on staff, including physicians and board members, a forty-hour program, MCMC University, which explores the key issues needed to implement the Planetree model. It has also instituted shared governance to empower nurses in decision making and has remodeled the entire facility to create a healing and homelike atmosphere. The remodeling includes a four-story atrium with a waterfall and baby grand piano in the lobby, as well as patient activity rooms and kitchens with dining areas on patient floors.

North Hawaii Community Hospital. Pat Linton, C.E.O., Box 2799, Kamuela, Hawaii 96743. Phone: (808) 885-2722. This hospital is in the planning phase of creating a healing village that incorporates healing architecture and grounds and holistic services. It plans to have an organic garden with medicinal herbs, a department of healing, and multiskilled practitioners with special training in healing methods as well as traditional methods. It is involving the community in planning and is exploring with complementary religious and ethnic groups the use of such methods as Kahuna healing, Buddhist meditation, prayer, and acupuncture.

Queen's Medical Center. Norna Irvine, Project and Systems Coordinator, 1301 Punchbowl Street, Honolulu, Hawaii 96813. Phone: (808) 547-4603. A 506-bed, acute-care, not-for-profit teaching hospital, Queen's major goal in operational restructuring is to provide holistic nursing and medical care that is sensitive to each patient's beliefs, values, and culture. Its nursing staff has refined a preference form that assesses patient choices for daily activities and educational materials. In addition, it is redesigning its patient units to include a family room with library, an entertainment center, and access to an outside balcony. Units will also include a kitchen and private consultation room. Alternative therapy consultants, pastoral care, and other hospital representatives have been involved in the design.

Reading Rehabilitation Hospital. Joseph F. Nicosia, Director of Pastoral Care, Reading Rehabilitation Hospital, Reading, Pennsylvania 19611. This hospital uses a "healing paradigm" as a framework to guide the healing process. By using this paradigm the hospital helps patients to heal by encouraging them to increase self-esteem, make choices, accept one's circumstances, look to the future, connect with others, assess accomplishments, and discover religious significance. The hospital uses a healing health care group to empower staff and design systems. Its New Life Center runs workshops, counseling sessions, retreats, and support groups, and is a source of reading material for patients, families, and staff. In support of the concept, the hospital measures outcomes with assessment tools based on treatment and diagnostic areas.

St. Charles Medical Center. Nancy Moore, Project Director of Healing Healthcare, 2500 Neff Road, Bend, Oregon 97701. Phone: (503) 382-4321. St. Charles Medical Center is developing a model healing health care organization by reforming services around patients and their needs, developing leadership styles that contribute to healing, and instituting services that enhance the healing environment. The patient-focused transformation includes all departments and patient care units, with the orthoneuro unit being the first to go on line. By May of 1993, all the patient care areas will be in the implementation phase and utilize models of care delivery. The implementation phase will evolve into continuous quality improvement. To further enhance the healing environment, the Center is developing a variety of integrated services, one of which is "Arts in the Hospital." This service includes volunteer graphic artists, who arrange rotating art shows and work as part of the cancer support groups, and performing artists, including musicians, story tellers, and poets. Other services include licensed massage therapists and humor services. A life-skills service focused on prevention and developing healthy life-styles for patients and staff is being implemented. Another service is the Life, Death, Transition Service, which assists patients and their loved ones through the dying process. To help with the transformation, St. Charles is developing healing health care facilitators and internal consultants to support managers and staff in healing themselves and their relationships. Efforts are also under way to enhance the hospital's role in the health of the community.

Saint Joseph's Hospital of Atlanta. Kathryn J. McDonagh, M.S.N., R.N., C.N.A.A., President, 5665 Peachtree Dunwoody Road NE, Atlanta, Georgia 30342. Phone: (404) 851-7120. This hospital actively engages in healing its community by using mobile vans to provide medical services to the poor and homeless. Funding comes from various sources.

St. Vincent Hospitals & Health Services. Lynne O'Day, Vice President of Operations, 2001 West 86th Street, Indianapolis, Indiana 46260. Phone: (317) 338-7078. This not-for-profit system with four hospitals includes 1,000 beds. St. Vincent began restructuring with its 629-bed tertiary-care Indianapolis Hospital. It has reorganized four units, decentralizing nurses' stations and reorganizing jobs to include for each unit a representative, a clinical manager, a care team of nurses and technicians, a support assistant, and a pharmacist. The physical structure was changed to add laboratory facilities, radiology examination rooms, and satellite pharmacies to each unit. Also, bedside terminals and "nurse servers" (cupboards with bedside supplies) were added to each patient room. It plans to extend restructuring throughout its system.

Starbright Pavilion. Kathleen Unger, C.E.O., 11878 La Grange Avenue, Los Angeles, California 90025. Phone: (310) 446-5305. This freestanding pediatric facility was designed under the guidance of Steven Spielberg, film director and producer. It incorporates radical breakthroughs in healing health care architecture for children, as it also serves as a play area and theme park.

Washoe Medical Center. Ardis Kinney, Vice President, Patient Services; Tom Lavin, Life Skills Director, 77 Pringle Way, Reno, Nevada 89520. Phone: (707) 328-4629. Washoe offers a patient-centered, holistic approach to care. It integrates the ontological approach of the ART of Living paradigm and high-tech nursing care on its integrated medical unit and its life-skills inpatient unit as well as in outpatient programs. Visual imagery, music, art, and group work are included.

References

Adamski, B. "The Integrated Medical Unit." Paper presented at the Healing Health Care Project symposium, Reno, Nev., 1990.

Allawi, S., Bellaire, D., and David, L. "Are You Ready for Structural Change?" *Healthcare Forum Journal,* July/Aug. 1991, pp. 39–42.

Ambers, M. T., Boyd, M. E., and Ray, J. L. "What a Healthcare Client Needs from a Designer." *Journal of Health Care Interior Design,* 1991, *3,* 53–62.

American Hospital Association. "Caring for Patients with Alcohol and Other Drug Problems." In *Management Advisory, Healthcare Delivery.* Chicago: American Hospital Association, 1990.

American Nurses Association, Division of Nursing Practice and Economics. *Unlicensed Assistive Personnel Fact Sheet,* April 1992.

Anderson, E. "Preoperative Preparation for Cardiac Surgery Facilitates Recovery, Reduces Psychological Distress, and Reduces the Incidence of Acute Postoperative Hypertension." *Journal of Consultation and Clinical Psychology,* 1987, *55*(4), 513–520.

Anderson, R. *Wellness Medicine.* Lynnwood, Wash.: American Health Press, 1987.

Anthony, S. (ed.). "Radical Redesign of Hospital Organization and Patient Care Management Is Outgrowth of Shared Leadership Approach at Irvine Medical Center (Case Study)." *Healthcare Productivity Report,* 1990, *3*(12), 1–8.

Anthony, S. (ed.). "Case Study: Patient-Focused Care at Bishop Clarkson Hospital." *Healthcare Productivity Report,* 1991, *4*(5), 1–7.

Baier, S. "Patient Perspective." *Journal of Healthcare Interior Design*, 1989, *1*, 13–19.

Barber, T. "Changing 'Unchangeable' Bodily Processes by (Hypnotic) Suggestions: A New Look at Hypnosis, Cognitions, Imagining and the Mind-Body Problem." In A. A. Sheikh (ed.), *Imagery and Healing*. Imagery & Human Development Series. New York: Baywood, 1984.

Beckham, J. D. "Tools for Staying Ahead in the Nineties." *Healthcare Forum Journal*, July/Aug. 1991, pp. 63–66.

Beecher, H. "The Powerful Placebo." *Journal of the American Medical Association*, 1955, *159*, 1602–1606.

Bellaire, D., and Sauter, G. "Restructuring St. Charles Medical Center Operations." Unpublished report presented to St. Charles's Steering Committee, April 1992.

Bennett, H. L. "Behavioral Anesthesia." *Advances*, 1985, *2*, 11–21.

Bennett, H. L. "Behavioral and Psychological Issues in Anesthesiology: Strategies for Humanizing the Process of Surgery." Paper presented at the Second National Conference on the Psychology of Health, Immunity, and Disease by the National Institute for the Chemical Application of Behavioral Medicine, Orlando, Fla., Dec. 1990.

Bennett, H. L., Benson, D. R., and Kuiken, D. A. "Preoperative Instructions for Decreased Bleeding During Spinal Surgery." *Anesthesiology*, 1986, *65*, A245.

Bennett, H. L., De Morris, K., and Willits, N. "Acquisition of Auditory Information During Different Periods of General Anesthesia." *Anesthesia and Analgesia*, 1988, *67*, 512.

Benson, H. *The Relaxation Response.* New York: Avon Books, 1975.

Benson, H., and Stuart, E. *The Wellness Book: The Comprehensive Guide to Maintaining Health and Treating Stress-Related Illness.* New York: Carol Publishing Group, 1992.

Benya, J. "Lighting for Healing." *Journal of Health Care Interior Design*, 1989, *3*, 55–58.

Bertakis, K., Roter, D., and Putman, S. "The Relationship of Physician Medical Interview Style to Patient Satisfaction." *Journal of Family Practice*, 1991, *32*(2), 175–181.

Bertalanffy, L. von. "Foreword." In M. Davidson, *Uncommon Sense.* Los Angeles: Tarcher, 1983.

Borysenko, M. "Psychoneuroimmunology: Where Mind and Body Meet." Paper presented at the National Institute for the Chemical Application of Behavioral Medicine, Orlando, Fla., Dec. 4–7, 1991.

Bressler, D. "Guided Imagery: An Intensive Training Program for Clinicians." Paper presented at the Institute for the Advancement of Human Behavior, Seattle, 1984.

Bridges, W. *Transitions: Making Sense of Life's Changes.* Reading, Mass.: Addison-Wesley, 1980.

Bruning, N. S., and Frew, D. R. "Effects of Exercise, Relaxation, and Management Skill Training on Physiological Stress Indicators: A Field Experiment." *Journal of Applied Psychology,* 1987, *72*(4), 515–521.

Carpman, R., Grant, M. A., and Simmons, D. A. *Design That Cares: Planning Health Facilities for Patients and Visitors.* Chicago: American Hospital Publishing, 1986.

Cheek, D. B. "Unconscious Perception of Meaningful Sounds During Surgical Anesthesia as Revealed Under Hypnosis." *American Journal of Clinical Hypnosis,* 1959, *1*(3), 101–103.

Chicago Health Executives Forum. *The Hospital of the Future: Can the Patient-Focused Model Really Work?* Report of the 1991 Task Force, Chicago Health Executives Forum, 1991.

Clements, M. "The Growing Crisis in Health Care." *Parade: The Sunday Oregonian,* Feb. 28, 1993, p. 4.

Cooper, M. J., and Aygen, M. M. "Transcendental Meditation in the Management of Hypercholesterolemia." *Journal of Human Stress,* 1970, *5*, 24–27.

Cousins, N. *Anatomy of an Illness as Perceived by the Patient: Reflections on Healing and Regeneration.* New York: Bantam Books, 1979.

Cox, H. "Verbal Abuse Nationwide, Part 2: Impact and Modifications." *Nursing Management,* 1991, *22*(3), 66–69.

Cross, R. "Picture Perception and Patient Stress: A Study of Anxiety Reduction and Postoperative Stability." Unpublished paper, Department of Psychology, University of California, Davis, 1990.

Curtin, L. "Signs of Things to Come." *Nursing Management,* 1992, *23*(7), 7–8.

Dai, B. "Etymology of Chinese Word for 'Crisis.'" *Voices,* 1970, *5*(1), 70–71.

Davidson, M. *Uncommon Sense.* Los Angeles: Tarcher, 1983.

Deal, T., and Kennedy, A. *Corporate Culture: The Rites and Rituals of Corporate Life.* Reading, Mass.: Addison-Wesley, 1982.

Di Matteo, M. R., and Hays, R. "The Significance of Patient's Perceptions of Physician Conduct: A Study of Patient Satisfaction in a Family Practice Center." *Journal of Community Health,* 1980, *6*(1), 18–34.

DiMotto, J. "Relaxation: Six Techniques You Can Teach to Your Patients, Incorporate into Your Care, and Use Yourself—Even When You Just Have Ten Seconds to Spare." *American Journal of Nursing,* June 1984, pp. 754–758.

Distasio, C. "Consultive Services: Guidelines for Cost-Effective Utilization." *Health Care Supervisor* (Aspen Publishers), 1988, *6*(4), 1–17.

"Doing the Right Thing." *Legacy Choices,* Fall 1991, p. 3.

Dossey, L. *Recovering the Soul: A Scientific and Spiritual Search.* New York: Bantam Books, 1989.

Egbert, L., and others. "Reduction of Postoperative Pain by Encouragement and Instruction of Patients." *New England Journal of Medicine,* 1964, *270,* 825–827.

Ethridge, P., and Lamb, G. "Professional Nursing Case Management Improves Quality, Access and Costs." *Nursing Management,* 1989, *20*(3), 30–35.

Evans, F. "Unraveling Placebo Effects: Expectations and the Placebo Response." *Advances,* 1984, *1*(3), 11–20.

Ferguson, M. *The Aquarian Conspiracy: Personal & Social Transformation in Our Time.* Los Angeles: Tarcher, 1987.

Ferguson, T. "Planetree: The Homey Hospital." *Medical Self Care,* Nov./Dec. 1988, p. 263.

Flower, J. "More Tools for the Nineties." *Healthcare Forum Journal,* July/Aug. 1991, pp. 58–62.

Freshley, C. "Virtual Reality." Message #: 317 Project, Healing Healthcare Network Computer Bulletin Board System. Brighton, Colo., 1991.

Friedman, E. "Ethics and the Quality of Care." *Healthcare Forum Journal,* July/Aug. 1991, pp. 13–15.

Gappell, M. "Hospice Facilities." *Journal of Healthcare Interior Design,* 1990, *2,* 77–87.

Garnett, S. "Tips: Telling Isn't Teaching." *Patient Education Update: News, Views and Resources in Health Education,* 1992, *7*(1), 3.

Geber, B. "Can TQM Cure Health Care?" *Training,* Aug. 1992, pp. 25–34.

Gerteis, M., Daley, J., Delbanco, T., and Edgman-Levitan, S. (eds.). *Through the Patient's Eyes: The Picker/Commonwealth Program for Patient-Centered Care.* San Francisco: Jossey-Bass, 1993.

Gilpin, L., and Nelson, K. "A Healing Environment: The Planetree Hospital Project at San Jose Medical Center." *Journal of Healthcare Interior Design,* 1991, *3,* 139–149.

Glaser, R., and others. "Stress Related Immune Suppression: Health Implications." *Brain, Behavior and Immunity,* 1987, *1,* 7–20.

Goldsmith, J. "The Reshaping of Healthcare." *Healthcare Forum Journal,* July/Aug. 1992, pp. 34–41.

Goldsmith, J., and Miller, R. "Restoring the Human Scale." *Healthcare Forum Journal,* Nov./Dec. 1990, *33*(6), 22–27.

Gomberg, F., and Miller, K. "Case Study: Focused Care Centers, Decentralization, Cross-Training, and Care Paths Define 'World Class Healthcare' at Florida's Lee Memorial." *Strategies for Healthcare Excellence,* 1992, *5*(3), 1–7.

Gordon, S. "Caring Means Curing." *Utne Reader,* Jan./Feb. 1993, pp. 77–83.

Grieco, A., and others. "Current Perspectives: Strategies to Promote Patient Self-Management, New York University Medical Center's Cooperative Care Unit: Patient Education and Family Participation During Hospitalization—The First Ten Years." *Patient Education and Counseling,* 1990, *15,* 3–15.

Guynes, D. "Physical Rehabilitation Centers." *Journal of Healthcare Interior Design,* 1990, *2,* 37–47.

Haggard, A. *Handbook of Patient Education.* Rockville, Md.: Aspen, 1989.

Hall, H. "Hypnosis and the Immune System: A Review with

Implications for Cancer and the Psychology of Healing."
American Journal of Clinical Hypnosis, 1982, *25,* 92–103.

Hall, J. "Child Health Care Facilities." *Journal of Healthcare Interior Design,* 1990, *2,* 65–70.

Hanrahan, T. "New Approaches to Caregiving." *Healthcare Forum Journal,* July/Aug. 1991, pp. 33–38.

Harman, W., and Hormann, J. *Creative Work: The Constructive Role of Business in a Transforming Society.* Indianapolis: Knowledge Systems, 1990.

The Healthcare Forum: Patient-Focused Healthcare Delivery. Front Royal, Va.: Healthcare Marketing Information and Resource Center, 1991.

Heidt, P. "An Investigation of the Effects of Therapeutic Touch on Anxiety of Hospitalized Patients." Unpublished doctoral dissertation, New York University, 1979.

Heidt, P. "Effect of Therapeutic Touch on Anxiety Level of Hospitalized Patients." *Nursing Research,* 1981, *30,* 32–37.

Henderson, J., and Williams, J. "Making It Happen: Ten Steps to Restructuring Patient Care." *Healthcare Forum Journal,* July/Aug. 1991a, pp. 50–53.

Henderson, J., and Williams, J. "The People Side of Patient Care Redesign." *Healthcare Forum Journal,* July/Aug. 1991b, pp. 44–49.

Heywood, S. "Bill Moyers Special." Message #: 3063, Healing Healthcare Network Computer Bulletin Board System, Brighton, Colo., 1993.

Honsberger, M. M., and Wilson, A. F. "The Effects of Transcendental Meditation upon Bronchial Asthma." *Clinical Research,* 1973, *21,* 278.

Horn, M. "Hospitals Fit for Healing." *U.S. News & World Report,* July 1991, pp. 48–50.

Hurley, T., III (ed.). "Placebo Effects Unmapped Territory of Mind/Body Interactions." *Investigations,* 1985, *2*(1), 4–11.

Inlander, C., and Weiner, E. *Take This Book to the Hospital with You: A Consumer Guide to Surviving Your Hospital Stay.* New York: Warner Books, 1985.

Jaffee, D. *Healing from Within.* New York: Alfred A. Knopf, 1980.

Jenna, J. "Toward the Patient-Driven Hospital, Part 1." *Healthcare Forum Journal,* May/June 1986a, pp. 9–18.

Jenna, J. "Toward the Patient-Driven Hospital, Part 2." *Health-care Forum Journal,* July/Aug. 1986b, pp. 52–59.

Jevin, R. "Enhancing Hope in the Chronically Ill." In R. Jevin, *The Psychology of Health, Immunity and Disease.* Mansfield Center, Conn.: National Institute for the Clinical Application of Behavioral Medicine, 1991.

Joiner, W. "Leadership for Organizational Learning." In J. Adams (ed.), *Transforming Leadership.* Alexandria, Va.: Miles River Press, 1986.

Kaiser, L. *Lifework Planning.* Brighton, Colo.: Brighton Books, 1989.

Kaiser, L. "Boulder Community Hospital, Planetree, Integrative Body Works, Neonatal Massage." *Healing Healthcare Network Newsletter,* 1991a, *2*(4), 3–7.

Kaiser, L. "Design Tip." *Healing Healthcare Network Newsletter,* 1991b, *2*(4), 2–9.

Kaiser, L. (ed.). *Healing Healthcare Network Newsletter,* 1991c, *2*(2).

Kaiser, L. "Healing Ourselves, Our Relationships, Our Community." Paper presented at the second annual Healing Health Care Project Symposium, Reno, Nev., 1991d.

Kaiser, L. "Something to Think About." Message #: 44, 45, 52, 76, 171, 203, 276, 413, Healing Design Board of Health Online computer bulletin board system, Brighton, Colo.: 1991e.

Kaiser, L. "Therapeutic Sound." *Healing Healthcare Network Newsletter,* 1991f, *2*(1), 1–6.

Kaiser, L. "Honoring Our Connection: Healing Ourselves, Our Relationships, Our Communities." Paper presented at the Third Annual Healing Health Care Project Symposium, Sacramento, Calif., 1992.

Kanter, R. *The Change Masters: Innovation and Productivity in the American Corporation.* New York: Simon & Schuster, 1983.

Kaplan, S., Greenfield, S., and Ware, J., Jr. "Assessing the Effects of Physician-Patient Interactions on the Outcomes of Chronic Disease." *Medical Care,* Mar. 1989, *27*(3), S110–S126.

Kellman, N. "History of Health Care Environments." *Journal of Health Care Interior Design,* 1989, *3,* 19–27.

Klagsbrun, J., and Lorman, C. "Training Volunteer Home Visitors in the Community." Paper presented at the Third National Conference on the Psychology of Health, Immunity, and Disease by the National Institute for the Chemical Application of Behavioral Medicine, Orlando, Fla., Dec. 4–7, 1991.

Knaus, W., Draper, E., Wagner, D., and Zimmerman, J. "An Evaluation of Outcome from Intensive Care in Major Medical Centers." *Annals of Internal Medicine*, 1986, *104*(3), 410–418.

Kobasa, S. C. "Stressful Life Events, Personality and Health: An Inquiry into Hardiness." *Journal of Personality and Social Psychology*, 1979, *37*, 1–11.

Kreitner, C. "Work Redesign." Message #: 2128 Main Conferencing Board, Healing Healthcare Network Computer Bulletin Board System. Brighton, Colo., 1992.

Krieger, D. "Therapeutic Touch: Two Decades of Research, Learning, and Clinical Practice." Paper presented at the Twentieth Anniversary of Council Grove Conferences Voluntary Controls Program: The Menninger Foundation, Topeka, Kans., April 4–8, 1988.

Krieger, D., Peper, E., and Ancoli, S. "Physiologic Indices of Therapeutic Touch." *American Journal of Nursing*, 1979, *79*(4), 660–662.

Kübler-Ross, E. Paper presented at the Life, Death, Transition Workshop. Vashon Island, Wash., 1992.

Kuhn, T. *The Structure of Scientific Revolutions.* 2nd ed. Chicago: University of Chicago Press, 1970.

Kurtz, R. *Body-Centered Psychotherapy.* Mendocino, Calif.: Life-Rhythm, 1990.

Larkin, D. "Therapeutic Suggestion." In R. Zahourek (ed.), *Clinical Hypnosis and Therapeutic Suggestion in Nursing.* Philadelphia: Grune & Stratton, 1985.

Lathrop, J. P. "The Patient-Focused Hospital." *Healthcare Forum Journal*, July/Aug. 1991, pp. 17–20.

Leebov, W. *Service Excellence: The Customer Relations Strategy for Healthcare.* Chicago: American Hospital Publishing, 1988.

Leebov, W., and Scott, G. *Healthcare Managers in Transition: Shifting Roles and Changing Organizations.* San Francisco: Jossey-Bass, 1990.

Leininger, M. "Care Facilitation and Resistance Factors in the Culture of Nursing." *Topics in Clinical Nursing* (Aspen Publishers), 1986, *8*(2), 3.

Lerner, M. "Informed Choice in Cancer Treatment." Paper presented at the Third National Conference on the Psychology of Health, Immunity and Disease, by the National Institute for the Chemical Application of Behavioral Medicine, Orlando, Fla., Dec. 4–7, 1991.

LeShan, L. *Cancer as a Turning Point.* New York: Bantam Books, 1989.

Levinson, B. W. "States of Awareness During General Anesthesia." *British Journal of Anaesthesia,* 1965, *37,* 544–546.

Lewis, T. *The Lives of a Cell.* New York: Bantam Books, 1974.

Linton, P. (ed.). *T.H.E. Newsletter: Total Healing Environment* (Yavapai Regional Medical Center, Prescott, Ariz.), 1991, *1*(2).

Loudin, A. "A New Approach to Health Care." *For the Record,* Feb. 1991, *3*(6), 3–8.

Lulavage, A. "RN-LPN Teams: Toward Unit Nursing Case Management." *Nursing Management,* 1991, *22*(3), 58–61.

Lynch, J. J. *The Broken Heart: Medical Consequences of Loneliness.* New York: Basic Books, 1979.

McDonagh, K. "Work Redesign Ideas." Message #: 309, 350, and 639 Project, Healing Healthcare Network Computer Bulletin Board System. Brighton, Colo., 1991.

McKahan, D. A. "A New Architecture for Healthcare." *Healing Healthcare Network Newsletter,* 1991, *2*(1), 3–6.

McManis, G., and Pavia, L., Jr. "Partnering—The Ultimate Alliance." *Healthcare Forum Journal,* Sept. 1991, pp. 17–23.

Macrae, J. *Therapeutic Touch: A Practical Guide.* New York: Knopf, 1990.

Malkin, J. "Creating Excellence in Health Care Design." *Journal of Healthcare Interior Design,* 1991, *3,* 27–43.

Manthey, M. "Practice Partnerships: The Newest Concept in Care Delivery." *Journal of Nursing Administration,* 1989, *19*(2), 33–35.

Manthey, M. "Practice Partners: Humanizing Healthcare." *Nursing Management,* 1992, *23*(5), 18–19.

Martin, D., Hunt, J., Hughes-Stone, M., and Conrad, D. "The Planetree Model Hospital Project: An Example of Patient as Partner." *Hospital & Health Services Administration,* 1990, *35*(4), 592–601.

Maslow, A. *Toward a Psychology of Being.* New York: Van Nostrand, 1968.

Meehan, M. "The Effects of Therapeutic Touch on the Experience of Acute Pain in Postoperative Patients." Unpublished doctoral dissertation, New York University, 1985.

Meyercord, W., and Smith, M. "Transforming Healthcare: The Deming Approach." Presentation by Quorum Health Resources, Nashville, Tenn., at Bend, Oreg., 1992.

Miller, J. "President's Column: Use of Unlicensed Personnel in Acute Care Settings." *Nurse Executive,* 1992, *1*(1), 1.

Mitchell, J., and Bray, G. *Emergency Services Stress: Guidelines for Preserving the Health and Careers of Emergency Services Personnel.* Englewood Cliffs, N.J.: Prentice-Hall, 1990.

Moffit, K. *The Healthcare Forum: Patient-Focused Healthcare Delivery, Case Study IV: Bishop Clarkson Memorial Hospital.* Front Royal, Va.: Healthcare Marketing Information and Resource Center, 1991. Audiotape.

Naisbitt, J. *Megatrends: Ten New Directions Transforming Our Lives.* New York: Warner Books, 1984.

Naisbitt, J., and Aburdene, P. *Megatrends 2000: Ten New Directions for the 1990's.* New York: William Morrow, 1990.

Nathan, J., Hudson, G., Strazis, C., and Gomberg, F. "Case Study V: Lee Memorial Hospital—The QUEST Approach." In *The Healthcare Forum: Patient-Focused Healthcare Delivery.* Front Royal, Va.: Healthcare Marketing Information and Resource Center, 1991.

Nightingale, F. *Notes on Nursing.* Philadelphia: Lippincott, 1946. (Originally published 1859).

Olds, A. R. "With Children in Mind: Novel Approaches to Waiting Area and Playroom Design." *Journal of Health Care Interior Design,* 1991, *3,* 111–123.

O'Leary, D. (pres.). *The Joint Commission AMH Accreditation Manual for Hospitals.* Vol. 1: *Standards.* Oakbrook Terrace, Ill.: Joint Commission on Accreditation of Healthcare Organizations, 1990.

O'Malley, J., and Llorente, B. "Back to the Future: Redesigning the Workplace." *Nursing Management,* 1990, *21*(10), 46–48.

O'Regan, B. "Placebo—The Hidden Asset in Healing." *Investigations,* 1985, *2*(1), 1–4.

Orme-Johnson, D. W., and Schneider, R. "Reduced Health-care Utilization in Transcendental Meditation Practitioners." Paper presented at the Conference of the Society for Behavioral Medicine, Washington, D.C., Mar. 1987.

Ornish, D. *Dr. Dean Ornish's Program for Reversing Heart Disease.* New York: Ballantine Books, 1990.

Ouchi, W. *Theory Z: How American Business Can Meet the Japanese Challenge.* New York: Avon, 1981.

Pascale, R. T., and Athos, A. G. *The Art of Japanese Management: Applications for American Executives.* New York: Warner Books, 1981.

Pasternack, S. "Redefining Patient Care." *Deaconess Magazine,* Winter 1992, pp. 13–17.

Pavia, L., Jr., and Berry, H. R. "Partnering Strategies and Tactics." *Healthcare Forum Journal,* Sept./Oct. 1991, pp. 24–27.

Payer, L. *Medicine and Culture.* New York: Penguin Books, 1988.

Pennebaker, J. *Opening Up.* New York: Avon Books, 1990.

Peters, T., and Waterman, R. *In Search of Excellence: Lessons from America's Best Run Companies.* New York: HarperCollins, 1982.

Pimm, J. "New Ways to Provide Crisis Intervention for Heart Surgery Patients." Paper presented at the Third National Conference on the Psychology of Health, Immunity, and Disease by the National Institute for the Chemical Application of Behavioral Medicine, Orlando, Fla., Dec. 4–7, 1991.

Pollock, S. "The Hardiness Characteristic: A Motivating Factor in Adaptation." *Advances in Nursing Science,* 1989, *11*(2), 53–62.

Porter-O'Grady, T. "OR Staff Make Own Decisions in Shared Governance Model." *OR Manager,* 1988, *4*(9), 1–6.

Pronsati, M. "Patient-Focused Care." *Advance: For Physical Therapists,* 1992, *3*(15), 4, 5, 42.

Quinn, J. *An Investigation of the Effects of Therapeutic Touch Done Without Physical Contact on State Anxiety of Hospitalized Cardiovascular Patients.* Dissertation Abstracts International, 1982. (University Microfilms # DA 82 26 788)

Randolph, G. "Therapeutic and Physical Touch: Physiological Response to Stressful Stimuli." *Nursing Research,* 1984, *33,* 33–36.

Roter, D., Hall, J., and Katz, N. "Patient-Physician Communication: A Descriptive Summary of the Literature." *Patient Education and Counseling,* 1988, *12,* 99–119.

Rowland-Morin, P., and Carroll, G. "Verbal Communication Skills and Patient Satisfaction: A Study of Doctor-Patient Interviews." *Evaluation & the Health Professions,* June 1990, *13*(2), 168–185.

Rubik, B. "Toward a Real Science of Life." *Noetic Sciences Review,* 1992, no. 24, p. 21.

Ryan, J. "The Changing American Hospital: Back to the Future." *Hospital Materiel Management Quarterly,* 1991, *12*(3), 1–5.

Samuel, M. *Management Mastership: Transforming Reactive Management into Proactive Leadership.* Orange, Calif.: IMPAQ Organizational Improvement Systems, 1991.

Samuel, M. "Catalysts for Change." *Total Quality Management,* Sept./Oct. 1992, pp. 198–202.

Sandrick, K. "Future Fears: Organized Medicine Faces Managed Competition." *Hospitals,* April 20, 1993, p. 34.

Sasenick, S. (ed.). "The Healing Environment Compendium." *Healthcare Forum Journal,* Sept./Oct. 1992a, pp. 41–48.

Sasenick, S. (ed.). "Operational Restructuring: 19 Pioneering Models (Compendium)." *Healthcare Forum Journal,* July/Aug. 1992b, pp. 43–62.

Scheuerman, J., and Smith, V. "Selecting a Healthcare Consultant, Part II: Developing the Request for Proposal." *Journal for Healthcare Quality,* Jan.-Feb. 1992, *14*(1), 14–16.

Scott, C., and Jaffe, D. "From Crisis to Culture Change." *Healthcare Forum Journal,* July/Aug. 1991, pp. 33–38.

Seligman, M. *Helplessness.* New York: W. H. Freeman, 1975.

Senge, P. *The Fifth Discipline: The Art & Practice of the Learning Organization.* New York: Doubleday, Currency, 1990.

Sibbet, D., and O'Hara-Devereaux, M. "The Language of Teamwork." *Healthcare Forum Journal,* May/June 1991, pp. 27–30.

Sigardson, K. "Why Nurses Leave Nursing: A Survey of Former Nurses." *Nursing Administration Quarterly,* July 1982, pp. 20–22.

Simonton, O. C., Simonton, S., and Creighton, J. *Getting Well Again.* New York: Bantam Books, 1978.

Sine, D. "Experience Key to Compliance-Consultant Choice." *Health Facilities Management,* July 1992, pp. 68–71.

Slee, V. "The Center for Knowledge Coupling." Unpublished paper, Center for Knowledge Coupling, New York, 1993.

Smith, M. "Transforming Healthcare: The Deming Approach." Paper presented at Quorum Health Resources, at Bend, Oreg., 1992.

Sobel, D. "Mind Matters: Is Clinical Behavioral Medicine Cost-Effective?" Paper prepared by Kaiser Permanente Medical Care Program, Oakland, Calif., 1992.

Speedling, E., and Rosenberg, G. "Patient Well-Being: A Responsibility for Hospital Managers." *Health Care Management Review,* 1986, *11*(3), 9–19.

Starbright Pavilion Foundation. "Starbright, Starbright, First Smile I See Tonight." *Healing Healthcare Network Newsletter,* 1992, *3*(1), 1–6.

Strasen, L. "Redesigning Hospitals Around Patients and Technology." *Nursing Economics,* July/Aug. 1991, *9*(4), 233–238.

Suchman, A., and Matthews, D. "What Makes the Patient-Doctor Relationship Therapeutic? Exploring the Connexional Dimension of Medical Care." *Annals of Internal Medicine,* 1988, *108,* 125–130.

Summers, J. "Take Patient Rights Seriously to Improve Patient Care and Lower Costs." *Health Care Management Review,* 1985, *10*(4), 55–62.

Taylor, S. "Hospital Patient Behavior: Reactance, Helplessness or Control?" *Journal of Social Issues,* 1979, *35,* 156–185.

Thomas, L. *The Lives of a Cell: Notes of a Biology Watcher.* New York: Bantam Books, 1974.

Thompson, W. I. *The American Replacement of Nature.* New York: Doubleday, 1991.

Toffler, A. *The Third Wave.* New York: Morrow, 1981.

Tonges, M. "Redesigning Hospital Nursing Practice: The Professionally Advanced Care Team (ProACT) Model, Part 1." *Journal of Nursing Administration,* 1989a, *19*(7), 31–38.

Tonges, M. "Redesigning Hospital Nursing Practice: The Professionally Advanced Care Team (ProACT) Model, Part 2." *Journal of Nursing Administration,* 1989b, *19*(9), 19–20.

Tonges, M. "Work Designs: Sociotechnical Systems for Patient Care Delivery." *Nursing Management,* 1992, *23*(1), 27–31.

Ulrich, R. "Effects of Interior Design on Wellness: Theory and

Recent Scientific Research." *Journal of Health Care Interior Design,* 1991, *3,* 97–109.

U.S. Congress, Office of Technology Assessment. *Unconventional Cancer Treatments, OTA-H-405.* Washington, D.C.: U.S. Government Printing Office, Sept. 1990.

U.S. Department of Health and Human Services Office of the Secretary. *Secretary's Commission on Nursing: Final Report.* Vol. 1. Washington, D.C.: U.S. Government Printing Office, 1988.

Vogler, J. "Birthing Centers." *Journal of Health Care Interior Design,* 1990, *2,* 121–126.

Wallis, C. "Why New Age Medicine Is Catching On." *Time,* 1991, *138*(18), 68–76.

Walton, M. *The Deming Management Method.* New York: Putnam, 1986.

Walton, M. *Deming Management at Work.* New York: Putnam, 1990.

Wann, M. "Patient's Kin Prove Adept as Adjunct Nurses." *Healthweek News,* Mar. 25, 1991, p. 9.

Weber, D. O. "Six Models of Patient-Focused Care." *Healthcare Forum Journal,* July/Aug. 1991, pp. 23–31.

Weisman, C. S., Alexander, C. S., and Chase, G. A. "Job Satisfaction Among Hospital Nurses: A Longitudinal Study." *Health Services Research,* 1980, *15*(4), 341–364.

Winston, M. "New Business Heroes." *Executive Excellence,* Oct. 1992, pp. 5–6.

Wright, L. "Family Therapy." Paper presented at the Family Therapy Workshop, Bend, Oreg., 1992.

Yavapai Regional Medical Center (Prescott, Ariz.). *T.H.E. Newsletter: Total Healing Environment,* 1991, *1*(1).

Zander, K. "Nursing Case Management: Strategic Management of Cost and Quality Outcomes." *Journal of Nursing Administration,* 1988, *18*(5), 23–30.

Zemke, R. "Healthcare Rediscovers Patients." *Training,* 1987, *24,* 40–45.

Index